Knock Out Headaches

Foreword by Dr. Seymour Diamond, National Headache Foundation

Gary Ruoff, MD

SpryPublishing
ideas to life

Spry Publishing LLC
2500 South State Street
Ann Arbor, MI 48104 USA
www.sprypub.com

Printed and bound in the United States.

10 9 8 7 6 5 4 3 2 1

Library of Congress Cataloging-in-Publication Data on file.

ISBN: 978-1-938170-02-7 (paperbook)
ISBN: 978-1-938170-08-9 (e-Book)

Disclaimer: Spry Publishing LLC does not assume responsibility for the contents or opinions expressed herein.
Although every precaution is taken to ensure that information is accurate as of the date of publication, differences of
opinion do exist. The opinions expressed herein are those
of the author and do not necessarily reflect the views of
the publisher. Spry Publishing LLC does not recommend or
endorse any specific tests, physicians, products, procedures,
opinions, or other information that may be contained in
this publication. The information contained in this book
is not intended to replace the professional advisement of a
patient's doctor regarding medical information, diagnosis, or
treatment.

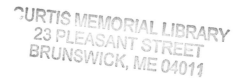

Dedication

I dedicate this to my loving wife Cynthia and
children Gary Stephen and Laura Anne
who supported me in my career in medicine.

I also wish to dedicate this book to the many wonderful
patients and headache sufferers throughout the nation.

Lastly, I'd like to acknowledge Robin Porter for her
editorial contributions to the book.

Foreword

It is indeed an honor to write this foreword at the invitation of my friend and colleague Gary Ruoff, MD. I have known Dr. Ruoff for many years, even before he began treating headaches, and have watched his evolution into one of the most proficient and compassionate physicians specializing in headache medicine. His knowledge has been fortified by his years of clinical research.

This book will not only be of great value to headache patients but will also serve as a resource to their families, friends, colleagues, and employers or teachers. This concise, well-researched, and knowledgeable book should be in the library of every headache patient.

Over the years, neurologists have come to dominate headache medicine. This was not always the case as internists, general practitioners, and other medical specialties were involved in the management of headache—and remain so. There is something special about this book. It is not only easily readable, but it is highly organized and an excellent source of information. It provides the patient with tools to successfully manage their problem. Above all, a book directed to headache patients should be written by an understanding and experienced primary care physician such as Dr. Ruoff.

I was asked to critique the manuscript and offer suggestions for improvement. While reading, I found little to add or detract. The explanations are simple yet thorough. The charts are easy to read and concise. Dr. Ruoff recognizes the value of a complete headache history and identifies the most valuable question in the patient interview—How many types of headache do you experience?

In 1973, Dr. Donald Dalessio and I published a book directed to all physicians who managed headache patients—*The Practicing Physician's Approach to the Difficult Headache Patient.* Our goal, throughout the first five editions of this textbook, was to produce simple and practical solutions to headache management for physicians of all specialties. In his book, Dr. Ruoff has successfully provided the headache patient with simple and practical information so that they can be advocates for their own care. He recognizes the role of the patient in dealing with the illness and how they can serve as a partner in headache management. This book is a welcome addition to the inventory of headache books.

Seymour Diamond, MD
Executive Chairman and Founder
National Headache Foundation
Chicago, Illinois

Table of Contents

Introduction

So you have headaches. Perhaps you've suffered from headaches for a number of years. When they first started, they may have only been a nuisance, easily controlled with over-the-counter (OTC) medications, or by simply "gutting it out" until the pain passed. Now, however, your headaches are occurring more often and are becoming more severe. Worse, the medications you relied on in the past are less effective or have become completely ineffective. Headaches may be interfering with your daily life—causing you to be less efficient at work, pass up social engagements, or miss out on family activities. Your headaches might be accompanied by sensitivity to light, sound, or even certain smells. Sometimes you may feel disoriented or light-headed. Your neck and shoulders may begin to tighten. What begins as a dull ache in your head intensifies as the hours pass, eventually developing into a "sick headache," which could include nausea and vomiting. Even the slightest motion of your head or body seems to make the headache more intense. At this point, all you want to do is find a dark room, crawl into bed, and stay there until the pain is gone.

If this sounds familiar, then you've picked up the right book. As a family physician for over 40 years, I've treated patients with a wide range of health issues. Over time, I developed a special interest in pain management, particularly for people suffering from chronic headaches. Eventually I became certified in headache treatment, but I never lost sight of what I found most gratifying as a family physician—the treatment of the *whole* patient. I don't treat just headaches; I treat *people* who suffer from headaches. When I first see a patient, I expect to spend an hour or more gathering information. I want to know *everything*, from family medical history and possible underlying health problems, to past success (or lack of success) with medications, as well as the patient's current stress level. I believe it takes time and a great deal of listening to make an accurate diagnosis and develop a successful treatment plan for any patient, especially those who have become frustrated or disheartened by a chronic condition, such as headaches.

Just as it is important for a physician to get to know the patient, I believe an informed patient is a good patient, and can be treated with more success. That's really what prompted me to write this book. The first step in treating any medical condition is to know what you're dealing with. Today, more than ever, information is readily available at a click of a button. However, medical data can often be confusing, contradictory, or even misleading. In addition, the sheer amount of information online can be overwhelming. It is my sincere hope that this book will help you make sense of this information, and arm you with the knowledge you need to control your headaches. It is not meant as a replacement for professional medical advice, but rather as a starting point for creating a dialogue with your doctor, as well as a resource for managing your headaches.

While I've helped patients with a myriad of health issues, including many life-threatening conditions, it is, most often, the headache sufferer who comes back to thank me for "giving me my life back." Why are headache patients so grateful? Because many of them have reached a point of surrender. They feel they have tried everything, exhausted all their resources, and still found no relief. Some of them have even been told that it's all in their heads (quite literally), and have sadly resigned themselves to living with chronic headaches. Perhaps you have also reached that point. If so, I urge you not to give up.

Headaches are not "curable." Alas, there is no magic formula or miracle drug. In fact, there is still much that is unknown about the causes and treatment of this often debilitating medical condition. There is no textbook way of treating headache patients. However, **headaches can be controlled and effectively managed.** With the right strategies—along with your willingness to do what's necessary—your quality of life can be dramatically improved. It won't be easy, but be assured, it can be done!

Together, we will explore the origin of headaches, their trigger mechanisms, and how you can manage them. Headaches are as individual as the people who suffer from them, and therefore must be treated accordingly.

We will take a look at how headaches can affect your state of mind; what role stress/anxiety plays; how to identify diet and lifestyle triggers; which underlying health issues could be contributing to your headaches; and what types of medications may be effective for your particular symptoms. And, because every patient provides a learning opportunity, you will also read about other headache sufferers, people just like you, who have found relief. It's comforting to know that headaches can be conquered.

One last note: as you read through the following pages, you will notice that there are many references to migraine. There is a reason for this. No matter its origin, any type of primary headache, when untreated, overly treated, or improperly treated, can increase in severity and/or frequency, leading to chronic headaches—and ultimately resulting in migraine symptoms, which require migrainous treatment. Even if you don't experience what you may think of as "classic" migraine symptoms (sensitivity to light and sound, nausea, dizziness), there's a very high probability that your headache is migraine. Migraine is, by far, the most common headache mechanism treated by physicians. And, just as the severity and duration of a headache can differ widely from person to person, so can the accompanying symptoms.

It's really up to you—the headache sufferer—to take control of your health and regain your life. Your primary care physician can provide you with the tools to manage your headaches, but only you can choose to use those tools properly. Becoming informed and actively assisting your doctor in your treatment is the key to obtaining relief from your pain. Let me help you take that first step. You have nothing to lose but your headache.

How To Use This Book

Don't simply read this book—put it to work for you. As you read, underline, highlight or circle points that pertain to you. Jot down notes to produce a quick reference sheet. Fill out the diaries. Put together the story of your personal headache complex. And use the checklist in Chapter 7 to track your progress. The book is designed to provide helpful hints for caring for yourself, as well as developing a treatment plan with your physician to get maximum benefits from the program I have outlined. Also, take advantage of additional references in the back of the book to further educate yourself on headache disorders. In other words, enlist all the resources you can to help knock out your headaches!

"A bad doctor treats symptoms; a good doctor treats ailments; but a rare doctor treats patients."

—Sidney J. Harris, American journalist, teacher, and lecturer

CHAPTER 1

Not All Headaches
Are Created Equal

Almost everyone has experienced an occasional headache. The term headache can be used to describe a wide range of discomfort, from a dull ache to pain so severe it renders a person helpless. Headaches can be a symptom of another medical condition (secondary) or exist on their own (primary). In addition, there are many types of specific headaches. However, when headaches are recurrent and interfere with daily activities, they are considered a *headache disorder,* which is the focus of this book. Although tension headaches are the most prevalent type of headache experienced, migraine is, by far, the most common type of headache treated by physicians. **Fully 95 percent of the headache patients I see in my practice are, in fact, migraine sufferers,** and in most cases, they are in a more advanced stage such that their way of life—their jobs, their social activities, or their family lives—is negatively affected. While much of this book and its references to research specifically address migraine, the fundamental cause of headache onset appears to be the same for all primary headaches.

Many people mistakenly associate migraine with a very specific set of symptoms—severe pain on one side of the head, accompanied by sensitivity to light and sound, dizziness, and nausea. In reality, we have come to learn that migraine can present itself in many forms: from mild discomfort to intense, throbbing pain; from diffuse to sharply focused; from a short-lived headache to one that lasts days, or even weeks. And it may or may not cause other symptoms. In other words, many headaches are migraines, but not all migraines are created equal.

Nobody Knows the Headaches I've Had

You are absolutely correct. It is difficult, if not impossible, for people who have never had a serious headache to understand what you are going through. As a headache sufferer, you've probably heard it all. Your spouse may ask, "Why can't you do the things you did in the past?" or "Why don't your medications work anymore?" Your children wonder why you're unable to attend school functions or sporting events. It's difficult for them to grasp why something as simple as playing outdoors is impossible for you when a headache strikes. Other people might be less sensitive and tell you to "Just get over it," or "It can't be that bad, just take an aspirin and go lie down." Even if you try to explain what you are feeling, they remain skeptical. They have no idea how debilitating an acute headache can be. Unfortunately, these types of comments or words of "advice" only add fuel to the fire by increasing your frustration and anxiety.

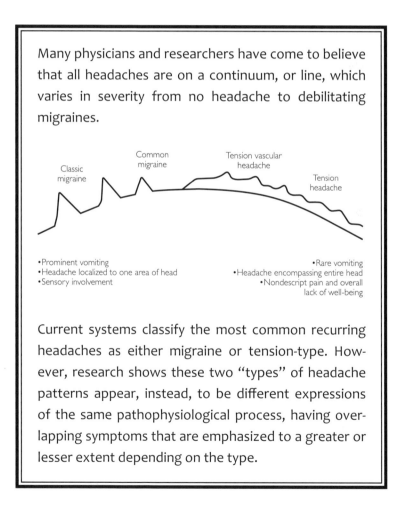

Many physicians and researchers have come to believe that all headaches are on a continuum, or line, which varies in severity from no headache to debilitating migraines.

Current systems classify the most common recurring headaches as either migraine or tension-type. However, research shows these two "types" of headache patterns appear, instead, to be different expressions of the same pathophysiological process, having overlapping symptoms that are emphasized to a greater or lesser extent depending on the type.

In fact, "frustrated" is a word I hear quite often from headache patients. And for good reason—headaches are very challenging to treat. Does this sound familiar? You've had headaches for many years. When they first started, you were able to control them with over-the-counter (OTC) medications, or your doctor may have even prescribed something to take for migraines. Over time, however, the medications became less effective, or no longer provided any relief. Eventually, your body became tolerant of these medications, and you either took an increased dosage or looked for alternatives.

It's also possible that the medication you were taking actually made the situation worse by causing what we call a "rebound headache"—when you stopped taking the medication, the headache came back even worse than it did before. Desperate, you may have even gone to an emergency room to get an injection to relieve your pain, only to be treated with disdain by the staff, who suspected you were a drug seeker.

Perhaps you have found that certain foods or beverages aggravate your headaches. That chocolate craving punishes you with pain, or your fondness for Chinese food leads to a splitting headache. And, forget about enjoying a glass of red wine or champagne, because you will certainly suffer the next day.

Of course you want an easy way out. You would like to have a pill that just takes care of the problem. After all, pills are used to effectively treat other ailments. The Internet is full of magic potions, and the pharmacy shelves are stocked with a wide variety of medications for migraine and "tension" headaches. Unfortunately, these often don't alleviate your symptoms, or may have helped for a while and then become ineffective. You have tried many approaches, but nothing seems to work. Not only are you becoming increasingly frustrated, but your doctor is as well.

As your headaches worsen, you begin to ask yourself, "Do I have a brain tumor or other serious condition such as an aneurysm or a stroke?" Perhaps a pinched nerve is causing all the neck pain and contributing to the pounding in your head? Could hormones or stress be the root cause of your headaches? Are certain foods the culprits? These are all good questions, and they, along with many other factors, must be investigated before a treatment plan can be developed specifically for your symptoms.

Part of the solution must rest with you. Other people may not "feel your pain," and your explanations might fall on deaf ears, but the best defense is still a good offense. Tell your detractors that you understand what they're saying—you don't like what your headaches are doing to you either. Assure them you are taking strong steps to successfully manage your headaches and return to your normal self. Ask them for their help and support in the process. And then, make a commitment to do it!

Headache management really comes down to four basic steps:

1. Educate yourself to the best of your ability about what is happening in your body, both physically and mentally.

2. Find a physician who is knowledgeable about your illness, who understands you as much as possible as a person, and with whom you can communicate openly and honestly.

3. Together, as a team, develop a total plan for headache management based on your unique symptoms and needs.

4. Commit to making the necessary changes outlined in the treatment plan.

This team approach is absolutely necessary for your eventual well-being. Keep in mind, however, that even with the best treatment plan, there will be bumps in the road to recovery. You may experience a bad day, or week, of headaches. Nonetheless, if you persevere, you will find the results tremendously rewarding, and wonder why it took you so long to begin the fight.

With that said, let's get started with the first step—education. I want you to become as knowledgeable as possible about your headaches, because an informed patient is easier to treat, and more likely to find relief.

"Could this be Alzheimer's?"

At age 23, Sally began to develop episodic migraine headaches. She had just graduated from college and was seeking employment in a very competitive job market. As hard as she tried, she could not find a job which fit her qualifications. After a year of intensive searching, she landed a managerial job that came with a lot of stress. Meanwhile, her husband was laid off from his job, and they had a young child to care for. The last thing she needed was to be incapacitated by headaches.

The pain in Sally's head was always on the right side. Over several years, the headaches became more severe and frequent, until she was having them three times a week. Along with the headaches, she had photophobia (sensitivity to light), phonophobia (sensitivity to sound), nausea, and eventually, vomiting. Even on a non-headache day, she didn't "feel right." Needless to say, she was feeling terrible most of the time. But what worried her most were some of her ancillary symptoms, such as dizziness and bouts of forgetfulness. Her grandmother had Alzheimer's Disease, and she was concerned that her forgetfulness could be an early indication of this disease. She also began to read up on brain tumors and became absolutely convinced she had something growing in her head.

After completing an in-depth medical history and physical examination on Sally, I assured her she wasn't suffering from Alzheimer's or a brain tumor. Though relieved to find she didn't have a life-threatening condition, she was still plagued by headaches, so we began a comprehensive treatment plan that included lifestyle modifications and other non-pharmacological remedies (see Chapter 4), as well as medication (see Chapter 5). Over time, we were able to get her headaches and associated symptoms under control, allowing Sally to get on with her busy life.

What, Exactly, Is a Headache?

Headaches are a very complicated subject. Even the medical community has yet to determine the root cause of migraine, and there is no specific medical test to determine the presence and severity of a headache. Rather, the diagnosis is made mostly on subjective information provided by you, the headache sufferer, along with the elimination of any other medical condition which might

---

Did You Know?
- Acute migraine is a common and often inadequately treated primary headache disorder.
- There are an estimated 30 million migraine sufferers in the United States.
- About half of these people are undiagnosed and "suffer in silence."
- Two-thirds of migraine sufferers are women.
- 18 percent of adult females and 6 percent of adult males suffer from migraine.

be the cause. That's why it's so important for you to become as knowledgeable as possible about your headaches, and form a partnership with your physician to determine the exact nature of your malady.

General Overview

Here is what we do know: migraine is a condition of the nervous system, which makes it a neurological disorder. People who suffer from headaches have inherited a very sensitive nervous system. This sensitive nervous system is passed on from generation to generation as a genetic trait, and causes the migraine-prone individual to process information differently. These individuals tend to be more sensitive to light, sound, tastes and smells, and their brains are generally more responsive to the activities going on around them.

Our nervous systems are stimulated by what we see and hear, what we taste and smell, what we touch and what touches us. In today's fast-paced, highly technological world, we are bombarded by stimulation! As stimuli increase, they become harder to control. Many of us lead rather hectic lives. We work harder and harder to fulfill our commitments, rush to meet deadlines, struggle to keep things organized, and find ourselves wishing for a 28-hour day to accomplish everything that needs to be done. For the migraine-prone individual, who processes stimuli differently and whose brain is highly-sensitive,

The Migraine Mechanism

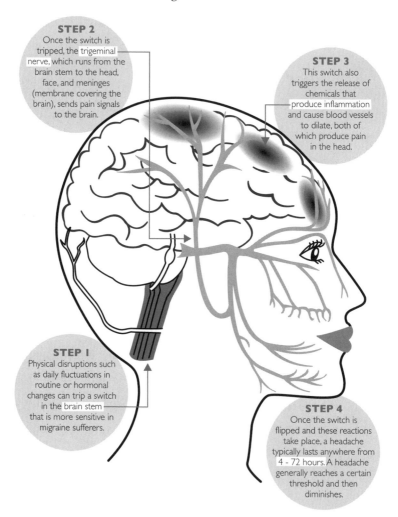

STEP 2
Once the switch is tripped, the trigeminal nerve, which runs from the brain stem to the head, face, and meninges (membrane covering the brain), sends pain signals to the brain.

STEP 3
This switch also triggers the release of chemicals that produce inflammation and cause blood vessels to dilate, both of which produce pain in the head.

STEP 1
Physical disruptions such as daily fluctuations in routine or hormonal changes can trip a switch in the brain stem that is more sensitive in migraine sufferers.

STEP 4
Once the switch is flipped and these reactions take place, a headache typically lasts anywhere from 4 - 72 hours. A headache generally reaches a certain threshold and then diminishes.

From Health Magazine *June 2012 (Ritzco)*

this onslaught is sometimes too much. The body and brain cannot adjust to the overload, and a headache begins.

The Migraine Mechanism

This is where things become a little tricky. There are multiple mechanisms responsible for the functional changes (pathophysiology) of a migraine, and medical research has yet to successfully define precisely how they work. While we all have the ability to get migraines—that is, the mechanisms are part of everyone's body—what activates these mechanisms and to what extent they are activated vary by individual. (For those brave folks who would like to delve deeper into the pathophysiology of migraine, refer to the sidebar on page 33.)

In the simplest terms, migraine causes swelling and inflammation of blood vessels around the head. More specifically, stimuli activate the trigeminovascular system, a group of nerve cells and tubes in the brain. The trigeminal nerves are the largest nerves in the head, while the term vascular refers to tubes which carry body fluids, such as blood and lymph. Therefore, a migraine actually affects the nervous system, the vascular system, and certain connective tissues.

During a headache, vessels and capillaries in the brain dilate or expand, while smooth muscles of the veins and arteries in the membrane surrounding the brain (dura) contract. Chemicals that influence neural activity or function, called neuropeptides, are released, resulting in inflammation or swelling. This inflammation further activates another nerve complex in the upper vertebrae, resulting in neck pain, which in turn sends signals to higher pain centers. The dura becomes hypersensitized to intracranial mechanical disturbances, causing further discomfort during physical activity. To make matters worse, the smallest nerves just under the skin on the same side of the body as the headache can become so hypersensitive that a feather touch might feel like you've been struck with a brick! This condition is called *ipislateral cutaneous allodynia,* which is thought to be a result of central trigeminal hypersensitivity.

If it sounds complicated, it is. Believe it or not, even this description is an oversimplification of a very complex process. Don't worry; it's not necessary for you to understand every detail of what happens during a headache—there won't be a quiz on Friday! However, it might help you to have a basic understanding of what is going on in your body during a headache. We will take a more in-depth look at migraine in Chapter 2, including the phases of migraine, what happens throughout the body (non-headache symptoms), and most importantly, migraine triggers and thresholds. For now, suffice it to say, a headache is much more than simply a pain in your head!

Even today, medical experts, including researchers, have differing opinions on the fundamentals of migraine attacks. There are many existing models of pathways that give rise to this debilitating condition, and many practitioners have dedicated their professional careers to the search for a solution. Much has been discovered over the years, all of which has assisted doctors in treating patients. Still, there is much left to learn.

Let's Review:

- Migraine sufferers are born with a highly sensitive nervous system.
- When this highly sensitive nervous system encounters a potential migraine trigger (or several triggers together), it sets off a complex process which causes swelling and inflammation of blood vessels in and around the head, resulting in a headache, and may also cause a variety of non-headache symptoms.
- What triggers the migraine mechanism, as well as the severity, duration, and accompanying symptoms, is different for everyone.

Making a Diagnosis

You might ask, "With all this going on in my head, and considering the conflicting medical theories, how is it possible to make an accurate diagnosis?" Often it is difficult. That's why I cannot emphasize enough the importance of patients being educated about their own symptoms.

First, you must realize the scope of the headache problem. The Headache Classification Subcommittee of the International Headache Society, to which nearly all practicing physicians adhere, recognizes no fewer than 300 types of headache. Obviously, we cannot list them all here, and quite frankly, that list would be of very little use to you. Most doctors will only encounter a small percentage of headaches on this list (perhaps nine or ten of them). Also, as I've stated before, the vast majority of patients I treat are migraine sufferers. However, in making a diagnosis, it's important to know some basics about how headaches are categorized.

Primary vs. Secondary Headaches

To start, all headaches can be divided into two broad categories: primary (benign) and secondary (worrisome). The distinction is usually not difficult. Primary or benign headaches are those which are not caused by structural problems or another disease. Fortunately, nearly all headaches, including migraines, fall into this category. When doctors evaluate a patient with headaches, they exclude "red flags" that may indicate another disease, and look for the following signs which support the diagnosis of a primary headache:

- History of previous similar headaches
- Family history of similar headaches
- Headaches connected to potential triggers such as certain foods and beverages, the menstrual cycle, or changes in weather
- Expected response to therapy
- Premonitory features (feelings that indicate a headache is starting) or aura followed by headache

Most worrisome to both the patient and the doctor is the secondary or organic headache. These headaches are caused by an underlying condition or disease, such as a brain tumor, an infection, or some type of head trauma. Because of the serious nature of these headaches, it is of the utmost importance that a physician rule out a secondary headache. Features associated with secondary headaches include:

- The onset occurs in a person older than 50 or younger than five years of age.
- There is a change in the headache pattern (increased frequency and/or severity).
- There is an onset of sudden "worst headache ever."
- A dull aching headache which progressively worsens over time and does not resolve.

- Exertion, coughing, sneezing, or sexual activity leads to the onset of headaches.
- There is a an unaccountable change in vital signs, such as fever, blood pressure, tachycardia (rapid heartbeat), anxiety, pallor, or sweating.
- Drowsiness, confusion, or memory impairment
- Slurred speech
- Ataxia (loss of coordination)
- Diplopia (abnormal papillary reflexes) or double vision
- Persistent tinnitus (ringing in the ears)
- The loss of the sense of smell
- Facial numbness, asymmetry (e.g., one eye not tracking like the other), or palsy
- Stiff neck, occipital (eye) pain, and tenderness
- Loss of hand grip power or tremor
- Motor and sensory loss in the extremities
- Loss of deep tendon reflexes
- Abnormal Babinski sign (a reflex movement in which the big toe turns upward instead of downward when the sole of the foot is tickled), or other neurologic signs
- Persistent headache following significant head trauma or whiplash injury
- Chronic cough, lymphadenopathy (abnormal enlargement of the lymph nodes), or weight loss
- History of malignancy, HIV, or other significant system disease

As noted, serious secondary headaches are rare, but they must be ruled out before any type of treatment plan is outlined.

From the Beginning

The first time you meet with a physician, preferably when you are not suffering from a headache, you may undergo a headache consultation. This is a more lengthy appointment than normal, and it will delve into your medical, family, and headache history, as well as your medications and treatments, dietary and sleeping habits, and other relevant lifestyle information. You may also be asked to submit to certain lab tests.

This data gathering serves two purposes. The first is for your physician to get to know you and for you to get to know him or her, and develop a rapport. The second reason is to establish a baseline, or level of "wellness," which will later be used as a comparison in treating not only your headache, but you as an entire person, rather than just a set of symptoms.

In Chapter 7, "The Patient-Doctor Partnership," we will talk more about how to prepare for that initial visit, including a list of helpful questions to ask yourself before you go.

One final note regarding diagnosis: often during a migraine episode, the body increases production of certain chemicals, sometimes called markers, which can be detected by a simple blood test. At this time, their presence cannot be used as a definitive diagnosis because the same chemicals are often produced during other inflammations which might be occurring in the body. They can, however, be compared to your baseline data to discern the degree of elevation and the possibility of migraine. This is as close to an affirmative diagnosis as is currently available.

Let's Review:

- Headaches can be primary (benign) or secondary (caused by an underlying disease or structural problem).
- Most headaches are primary, but secondary headaches must be ruled out before developing a treatment plan.
- At your initial visit, or headache consultation, be prepared for a long session of data gathering and possibly lab tests.

Before we dive deeper into the mysteries of migraine, I want you to know that while headaches are not curable they can be controlled, sometimes only requiring a change in lifestyle. And although many headache sufferers understandably feel as though the pain is "killing them," I can assure you that primary headaches are not life-threatening, nor is there any evidence that they may shorten your normal lifespan. As you read on, remember it's the *quality* of your life that is being treated, not merely your symptoms.

The Pathophysiology of Migraine

(Warning: The following description contains lots of complicated medical jargon! It is intended for the die-hard reader who wants to know the full story. If you feel a headache coming on while reading this, please stop immediately, and go and enjoy a non-caffeinated beverage!)

You might ask, "What is 'pathophysiology'?" If it sounds Greek to you, you're right. The word comes from two Greek terms: patho, meaning suffering, and physiology, meaning the function of living organisms. In medicine, it has come to mean the functional changes that accompany a particular syndrome or disease.

Multiple physiologic mechanisms are responsible for the pathophysiology of migraine. Triggers such as stress or trauma, odors, changes in sleep pattern, or specific foods or drugs activate the trigeminovascular system— a system of nerves and tubes in the head. Trigeminal neurons release vasodilatory (blood vessel-dilatory) and inflammatory neuropeptides (chemicals that influence neural activity), of which calcitonin gene-related peptide (CGRP) appears to be the most important in migraine. Intracranial vessel dilation and protein extravasation (a process in which blood is forced from a vessel into surrounding tissue) in the dura mater result in neurogenic inflammation (swelling) that further activates the trigeminocervical complex, which sends signals to higher pain centers.

Along with the release of CGRP, a decrease in serotonergic neural transmission (serotonin) has been implicated in the pathophysiology of migraine. Serotonin (5-HT) regulates the vascular smooth muscle tone of meningeal blood vessels via 5-HT receptors, which causes vasoconstriction. In addition, 5-HT has inhibitory effects on trigeminal nerves that synapse onto the dural vessels, and brainstem trigeminal nuclei via the 5-HT receptor. Further credibility is lent to this model by studies which show that magnoencephalographic imaging reveals brain stem activity in patients suffering from migraine attacks as opposed to non-migraine pain. The trigeminal nerve and other cervical nerves are thought to stimulate the vascular reaction of migraine described above.

During migraine, mechanosensitive nociceptors (receptors for painful stimuli) in the dura become hypersensitive to intracranial mechanical disturbances, which may cause an increase in pain during physical activities. Sensitization of central trigeminal afferents (i.e., second-order trigeminal neurons) can also occur during migraine. Cutaneous allodynia involving the side of the body ipsilateral to the headache side in migraine has been proposed as a manisfestation of central trigeminal hypersensitivity, and in one study it was found that 79 percent of 42 migraine sufferers included in the analysis demonstrated ipsilateral cutaneous allodynia during migraine.

Yet another model asserts that during a migraine episode, the trigeminal cervical nucleus in the descending tract of the trigeminal nerve interacts with sensory fibers from the upper cervical roots. This convergence of sensory pathways allows the bidirectional referral of painful sensations between the neck and sensory receptive fields of the face and head, and may be responsible for the referral of cervical pain to the head. Consequently, neck pain, muscle tension, and cervical muscle tenderness are common and prominent symptoms of primary headache disorders. Whew!

Chapter 2
Understanding Migraine

Why Me?

One of the questions I hear frequently from headache sufferers is "why me?" It's natural to feel frustrated, or even victimized, by chronic headaches, especially if you have been living with them for a long period of time. As we discussed in Chapter 1, the simplest answer to that question is that you have inherited a sensitive nervous system, which can be easily overloaded and lead to a migraine. In other words, you are wired that way. Headaches occur when your nervous system is overstimulated by a potential migraine trigger, or more often several triggers that occur together.

Because this tendency runs in families, you may have a relative or several relatives who also suffer from migraines. While you can't change the genetic trait you were given, you can learn to control it. So, instead of asking "why me?" the important questions should be: what triggers my headaches, and what can I do to prevent them? Instead of feeling like a helpless victim, you can learn to fight back.

Triggers and Thresholds

Two of the most important concepts in headache management are thresholds and triggers. Each headache patient has a threshold for particular triggers, and when that threshold is exceeded a headache will occur. Let's use the example of a glass of water—the threshold is the top of the glass and the water represents potential migraine triggers. As long as the water doesn't reach the top of the glass, it will not spill over. However, if you keep pouring water into the glass, you will eventually reach the point of overflowing, causing a headache.

What are those triggers? Just as the symptoms, duration, and severity of headaches are different for everyone, so are the triggers or combination of triggers. Potential migraine triggers come in many forms, including:

- Environmental factors, such as changes in weather or altitude
- Hormonal fluctuations
- Sensory stimuli, such as perfume, tobacco smoke, flickering lights, and loud noises

- Changes in habits, such as sleep patterns and work schedule
- Stress or other emotional crisis
- Some medications, including painkillers
- Certain foods and drinks

The charts on the following pages provide a more complete list of potential migraine triggers. However, **the most common triggers are dietary.** The four main dietary triggers I see in migraine patients are caffeine, chocolate, monosodium glutamate (MSG), and certain artificial sweeteners. Here are some others:

Caffeine	Coffee, decaf coffee, tea (hot and cold), and soda.
Chocolate	Milk and dark chocolate specifically.
Nuts	Avoid all varieties of nuts.
Certain Fruits/ Juices	Citrus fruits and juices, bananas, and dried fruits including raspberries, plums, papayas, passion fruit, figs, dates and avocados.
Certain Vegetables	Especially onions, sauerkraut, pea pods, and some beans including broad Italian, fava, navy, and lentils. Allowed are garlic, shallots, spring onions, leeks, and scallions.
Cheese/Dairy Products	Aged cheeses are the worst. Allowed are cottage cheese, ricotta, cream, and high-quality American. Avoid pizza, yogurt (frozen and non-frozen), sour cream, and buttermilk.

Yeast-Risen Baked Goods	Homemade or restaurant-baked breads, sourdough, bagels, doughnuts, pizza dough, soft pretzels, and coffee cake.
Alcohol/Vinegar	Red wine, champagne, and dark-colored, heavy cocktails. Limit ketchup, mustard, and mayonnaise usage.
Processed Meats and Fish	Any meats preserved with nitrates or nitrites, including hot dogs, sausage, salami, pepperoni, bologna, liverwurst, beef jerky, ham, bacon, patês, smoked/pickled fish, anchovies, and caviar. Any meats containing tyramine like beef and chicken livers, and wild game. Any meats that are aged, marinated, smoked, canned, cured, tenderized, or fermented.
Monosodium Glutamate (MSG)	Found in ready-to-eat meals, processed foods, some seasonings, low-fat, low-calorie foods, Chinese (and other) restaurant foods, soups and bouillons, veggie burgers, and protein concentrates.
Aspartame	Nutrasweet. Sweet' N Low (saccharin) may also be a trigger. Allowed: Splenda (sucralose).
Other possibilities	A cultured or fermented soy product, like miso and tempeh, or highly-processed soy protein concentrates.

Adapted from, "Heal Your Headache: The 1-2-3 Steps to Healing Your Pain," D. Buchholtz, Workman Publishing © 2002

Is Your Glass Half Full?

Now, you may be saying, I don't get a headache every time I eat chocolate or drink coffee, or Chinese food doesn't really bother me. That may be true, because **often it's not simply one trigger that causes a headache, but the combination or cumulative effect of several.** Let's go back to our glass of water example. Normally, having a "glass half full" is a positive thing, but in headache management it's a cautionary sign. On any given day, you may have a glass of water that is already half full due to unavoidable factors such as rising heat and humidity, the lack of sleep, or increased stress over a big project at work. Then, you add more "water" to that glass in the form of a soda with caffeine, or a diet soda loaded with artificial sweetener. This combination of triggers cause the water to reach the top of the glass and spill over the sides, and you end up with a headache.

The whole idea here, and I can't stress this point enough, is that **you must decrease the number of triggers or risk factors in order to successfully manage migraines.** A patient who identifies and decreases his or her potential triggers can often manage migraines without medication, or with minimal use of medication. At the beginning of a patient's treatment plan, I often recommend eliminating more triggers than necessary, and then as the patient's headaches resolve, he or she can gradually add foods or drinks back into the diet (one at a time) to identify the real culprits.

There are many triggers that are unavoidable or difficult to avoid, so the trick becomes steering clear of the triggers you can control, which most often are dietary. So, for example, you don't want to indulge in your favorite chocolate treat or a large latte on a day when there is a thunderstorm, because the change in barometric pressure is already a potential trigger. You can't control the weather, but you can control what you eat or drink. A person with a tendency toward migraine has an increased sensitivity to smells such as perfume or smoke, flickering lights, and loud noises. It can be difficult to avoid perfumes in a store or smoke in a public place, or you may enjoy going out to listen to loud music once in a while. If you can't escape the situation, just make sure you don't make it worse.

We'll take a closer look at how to identify your particular triggers by keeping a headache diary, as well as provide a detailed migraine diet later in the book. For now, suffice it to say, identifying and avoiding potential triggers can be a one-two punch for knocking out headaches.

Let's Review:

- Every migraine patient has a threshold for particular triggers or combinations of triggers. When that threshold is exceeded, the result is a headache.
- It is often the combination or cumulative effect of several triggers that causes a headache.
- Identifying and avoiding potential migraine triggers is key to successful headache management.

Potential Headache Triggers

Diet

Alcohol (red wine and champagne)

Chocolate

Caffeine

Aged cheeses

Monosodium glutamate (MSG)

Aspartame (Nutrasweet)

Nuts

Nitrates

Hormones

Menstrual cycle

Ovulation

Hormone replacement (progesterone)

Sensory Stimuli

Strong light or flickering lights

Odors (perfume, smoke)

Loud noises

Stress
Letdown following stressful periods
Times of intense activity
Loss or change (death, separation, divorce, job
    changes, moving)
Crisis

Changes in Environment or Habits
Weather (rise or fall in barometric pressure)
Travel (crossing time zones)
Seasons
Altitude
Schedule changes
Sleeping patterns
Dieting, skipping meals, erratic meal schedule
Irregular physical activity

Medications
Contraceptives, including birth control pills,
    medroxy-progesterone injections (Depo-
    Provera), and levonorgestrel implants (Norplant)
Hormone replacement therapy
Adrenaline-like drugs, stimulants and diet pills,
    including:
        Bronchodilators for asthma (e.g., Proventil,
            Serevent)
        Over-the-counter stimulants (e.g., No-Doz)
            and herbal stimulants
        Methylphenidate (Ritalin, Concerta)
        Dextroamphetamine (Adderall, Dexedrine)

OTC diet pills

Prescription diet pills (e.g., Ionamin, Meridia)

Vasodilators, such as:

    Nitrates for heart disease (e.g., Isordil, Nitro-Dur)

    Sildenafil citrate (Viagra)

Others

    Isotretinoin (Accutane) for acne

Selective serotonin reuptake inhibitors (e.g., Prozac) and buproprion (Wellbutrin) for depression

"I hate Mondays!"

Ann works hard all week. She has a high-pressure job with tight deadlines, which makes her work environment very stressful. By the time Friday arrives, she is ready to let off a little steam and relax. But, after what is supposed to be a nice, relaxing weekend, she often wakes up on Monday morning with a severe headache. What is going on?

This is a fairly common occurrence, which we refer to as the "Monday Morning Headache," although it sometimes occurs on Sunday, as well. Patients will notice a pattern of headaches occurring at the end of the weekend. As if Mondays aren't hard enough, they find themselves suffering with a migraine.

First of all, the "letdown" after a particularly stressful work week can trigger a headache on its own. But more often, it is a combination of factors that happen over the weekend that results in a migraine. TGIF! Many of us celebrate the end of the workweek by going out and having a few drinks, such as red wine or a favorite cocktail. This was the case with Ann, who liked to join friends for a couple of glasses of wine after work. Then, after staying up later than usual, Ann liked to sleep in on Saturday. She often spent Saturday and Sunday rushing around trying to complete all her errands, instead of finding time to relax. To keep herself going, she fueled herself up with more coffee than she usually drank during the week, setting herself up for a caffeine withdrawal. By the time Monday morning arrived, Ann would develop a nasty headache that grew increasingly worse throughout the day.

Because Ann is prone to migraines, the combination of wine, change in sleep patterns, and increase in caffeine fills her "water glass" to overflowing, particularly if there are other environmental or hormonal factors occurring at the same time. Fortunately for Ann, we were able to manage her headaches with simple lifestyle and dietary changes.

Having fun on the weekend is certainly advisable. However, if you are prone to migraines, you need to be aware of the triggers that tend to happen on those days off. Try to limit the amount of alcohol you drink, stick to regular sleep/wake patterns as much as possible, avoid or ideally eliminate caffeine, and find some time to relax and participate in activities you enjoy.

Phases of the Migraine

It would be nice if headache sufferers had a built-in gauge that lets them know when they are reaching their threshold. Then, a warning signal would go off, and you would be alerted to avoid potential triggers. While your body may not have this handy gauge, you can become more attuned to the onset of a migraine by knowing the symptoms that often precede a headache, along with the phases of a migraine. Patients who are able to pinpoint the changes occurring in their bodies can often prevent or reduce the severity of a headache.

Migraine is not only a headache, but a complete symptom process which affects the whole person. The entire body is being overwhelmed by the hyper-excitability of the nervous system, which is why there are many non-headache symptoms that can accompany a migraine. These symptoms are unique to each individual, but migraines can be divided into three phases: premonitory (symptoms that appear before the headache begins); symptoms that occur with the headache; and postdromal (symptoms that persist after the headache resolves).

Premonitory Symptoms

You may not be able to predict the future, but many people can foresee the onset of a migraine. A few minutes to 24 hours before a headache, you might experience premonitory symptoms (sometimes referred to as the prodrome). These may include fatigue, irritability, difficulty concentrating, and sensitivity to light or sound. Muscle pain, especially in the neck and shoulders is also common. Some patients experience a loss of appetite, while others crave certain foods. You may also feel anxious or depressed. It's also possible that none of these problems occur before your headache. However, studies show that 50–70 percent of migraine sufferers are aware of these pre-headache signs.

Recognizing these symptoms will give you a chance to reverse the process before it actually begins. For instance, by removing yourself from a stressful situation, resting or taking a short nap, or using a mild OTC medication, you may be able to prevent a full-blown migraine. Unfortunately, many people do the opposite. When they feel a headache coming on, they begin to work harder and faster in an attempt to get everything done before the headache worsens, or tense up and become more anxious anticipating the pain to come. By adding more stress, you are almost guaranteeing that your headache will be a bad one. Instead, consider these premonitory symptoms as a warning sign and take steps to help yourself.

Auras

About 15–25 percent of the time, patients develop an aura before a headache. An aura is a dramatic experience that happens when the metabolism in certain tissues of the brain is decreased. There are several types of aura, but the most common happens in the area of the brain that controls vision. You may see flashing lights, zigzag patterns of light and dark, or spots in your vision. They might be black and white, or they may be quite colorful. These light auras usually move across the visual field, from right to left, or left to right. What's interesting is that if you close your eyes, you can still see the pattern, as if it's imprinted on the inside of your eyelids. That's because the light show is happening in your brain and not your eyes.

Auras can also involve sound. Patients who experience a sound aura describe it as a roaring freight train. Less common are taste auras, in which you have a bitter taste in your mouth. Finally, you may develop *paresthesia*, which is tingling or numbness around the face, arms or legs.

Auras can be unique. I took my grandchildren to the play *Alice in Wonderland*, which featured distorted figures (think of the Mad Hatter with his abnormally large head) and bright, colorful costumes. It reminded me of a patient who described seeing a similar scene as a prelude to his migraine. (Interestingly, the author of *Alice in Wonderland*, Lewis Carroll, did have migraines and saw these distorted figures in his auras.)

Fortunately, most auras resolve without any special treatment. They typically begin about 30 minutes to an hour prior to the headache and only last that long. In some rare cases, auras can be permanent. This is usually the result of another problem in the brain, which requires separate treatment. While they can be very disturbing to the patient, auras are not medically alarming.

Headache Phase

Despite your best efforts, you may not be able to ward off a headache. When a headache starts, it sometimes feels as though it comes in waves. If the headache begins as mild, this is the best time to take medication for its treatment. This may be an OTC painkiller or something prescribed by your doctor. Migraines will sometimes resolve when they are caught in a mild state. If let go, the headache typically progresses from mild to moderate and then severe. At this point, it becomes much more difficult to treat, and many medications will not work properly. Therefore, treating a headache early improves treatment response.

Headaches usually develop gradually. Sometimes it's difficult for patients to determine exactly when a headache begins. You may become aware of slight pressure in your head rather than pain, or the muscles in your neck and around your head could feel stiff and tender. Some patients experience stuffiness in their nasal passages. This congestion often misleads people into thinking they are having a sinus problem instead of a migraine, when in fact it's the migraine mechanism causing the inflammation. This mild phase can last anywhere from several minutes to many hours.

As the headache progresses, the pain becomes more severe and localized, usually behind one eye or across the forehead. While migraines can cause pain in any part of the head, they most commonly occur on one side of the head, which may begin to throb or pulsate with pain. This is typically the point at which most patients recognize they are getting a migraine. Often what begins as a simple headache, which you suspect is a tension or sinus headache, develops into a classic migraine.

In the moderate-to-severe headache phase, the nerves on the outside of the brain become more sensitive. This is called *peripheral sensitization*, and it's characterized by throbbing pain that gets worse with activities. Even mild exertion, such as coughing or sneezing can cause intense pain. Once the nerves outside the brain become sensitized, they bombard the brain's internal nerves with pain signals. This *central sensitization* causes signals from the brain that normally would not be painful to become highly sensitive. Even touching a patient at this point might cause discomfort. Normal light, sound, tastes, and scents may become intolerable. Non-headache symptoms such as nausea and vomiting, diarrhea, nasal congestion, and even anxiety or sadness can also occur. Finally, the migraine sufferer has no choice but to seek refuge in a dark, quiet room. This stage of the migraine may last 24 to 48 hours, and treatment may be difficult.

Postdrome or Post-Headache Phase

As if having a headache wasn't bad enough, many migraine sufferers often experience a postdrome or post-headache phase once the headache resolves. Symptoms of this phase include fatigue, muscle aches, irritability, loss of appetite, and mood changes, such as depression. We refer to this phase as the "migraine fog," because many people describe this period as feeling "not quite right," or "walking around in a fog," unable to focus or think clearly. Many patients will wake up with a "heavy head," which persists all day, or experience flu-like symptoms. I have had patients tell me they feel as though the energy has been sapped from their bodies. It becomes difficult to perform daily tasks, and you may even experience a severe case of the "blahs." At times, this phase can be just as disabling as the headache itself. Unfortunately, this migraine fog can persist for another 24 to 48 hours, depending on the individual.

So, if you add together up to a day of premonitory symptoms, a day or two of headache, and another day or two of postdrome symptoms, you can be affected by a migraine for three to five days. The overall impact of a migraine can result in your being out of commission for several days, or even a week. That's why it's so important to understand the full story of your headaches. The goal is not to simply treat the symptoms, but to take control of the entire process.

Again, the use of a migraine diary is very helpful in determining the phases of your headaches. Do your headaches typically begin in the morning or the afternoon? Do they start out mild and progress over minutes or hours? What warning signs or signals do you experience? What symptoms do you feel at each phase? All of this information will make it easier for you and your physician to design a treatment program.

What's Your Baseline?

Everyone has a health baseline. This is where you are feeling good and energetic, functioning properly without a headache or other symptoms. A physician needs to determine your baseline in order to determine your headache patterns and develop treatment options. With migraine, this baseline can change.

By definition, migraine is a headache that recurs over time. Thankfully, for many patients, migraine attacks are infrequent, and once the headache resolves, they return to their baseline or normal functioning. However, sometimes occasional headaches, if left untreated, can become more frequent and even daily occurrences. This means your baseline has been altered and needs to be adjusted. Even when there is no headache present, patients complain of not feeling right. They often have mild headaches or feel fatigued and achy all the time. This is called *migraine transformation* and leads to a diagnosis of chronic migraine. Ironically, the overuse of medication used to treat occasional migraine can lead to chronic migraine.

Think of a six-cylinder motor in your car. If one of the cylinders malfunctions and there are only five cylinders working, your car will still take you where you want to go. But the engine is running rough, the car is going more slowly than you would like it to, and it's definitely not up to peak performance. That's how chronic

---

Let's Review:

- Migraine is more than a headache. It evolves in stages over hours and possibly days, and can include many non-headache symptoms.
- Identifying the phases of your headache, especially premonitory symptoms, can help you prevent or lessen the severity of a migraine.
- When you feel a headache coming on, take steps to protect your nervous system—remove yourself from stressful situations, practice relaxation techniques, take a walk, or get some rest.
- Keeping a headache diary can help your doctor determine patterns and develop more effective treatments.

migraine affects people during the pre-headache and post-headache phases. They never feel as though they are performing on all six cylinders.

Avoiding this chronic problem is very important since it becomes extremely difficult to treat effectively. We will discuss many non-pharmacologic strategies, along with the proper use of medications, later in the book to help control your headaches, as well as prevent a chronic pattern. In the meantime, remember that decreasing the sensitivity of the nervous system and reducing its triggers is the key to successful headache management.

"She's usually such a dynamo."

Sara is a 55-year-old nurse, and most people would describe her as a dynamo. She is usually cheerful and friendly, willing to help both patients and the physicians with any task. Patients love her because she often goes the extra mile to assist them. Unfortunately, she also suffers from migraines two to three times per month, which takes her out of the office for several days at a time. These headaches are followed by a migraine fog.

As soon as I see Sara come into the office after a headache, I know she is suffering from a migraine fog. Her eyes are glassy and have a distant look. Her comprehension is much slower. She is more irritable and becomes annoyed at the phone which is constantly ringing. With a pen in one hand and the telephone in the other, trying to take a message while the physician is barking out an order as he passes by, she would, I can tell, like to scream. Usually she can easily handle three or more tasks at once, without complaint. But in a migraine fog, she will often become teary-eyed and leave the desk to compose herself. This cycle of anxiety and stress, feeling that she is being pushed all day and overwhelmed, makes matters worse.

Fortunately, this migraine fog can be resolved with the same migraine-specific medications used to treat the headache (see Chapter 5), even when no headache is present. Some migraine fogs respond better than others to treatment, so it may take some trial and error. When a medication is effective, it will dissipate a migraine fog within an hour. It's important for Sara to take her medication as soon as she wakes up with the symptoms, and not wait and see if they will go away on their own.

When migraine fogs do not respond to medication, just like migraines themselves, it's time to reassess your situation. Are you getting enough sleep? Are you eating three meals a day and not skipping meals? Are you doing neck exercises to lessen the tension that can build there? Are you finding ways to relax and manage stress? Are you avoiding your migraine triggers? In Sara's case, because she is such a dynamo, and has so many demands on her time, it's important for her to put these demands in perspective, as well as following her prescribed treatment. It's all part of the big picture.

Migraine in Children

Since headaches are hereditary, you may be concerned about your children developing migraines. Diagnosing migraines in children can be tricky because they often have a different presentation of symptoms than adults. In fact, you and your doctor may not initially recognize these symptoms as migraine. While some children will have severe headaches, others experience a variety of non-headache symptoms that masquerade as other problems. Children may start off with periodic syndromes that are commonly precursors to migraine, including cyclic vomiting, abdominal migraine, and non-paroxysmal vertigo of childhood.

Cyclic severe vomiting or recurrent vomiting: A young child with migraine may have attacks of severe nausea and vomiting. What makes this baffling is that there is usually no abdominal pain, and there is a complete resolution of symptoms between attacks. The intense nausea and vomiting may last from one hour to five days. During these attacks the patient vomits at least four times per hour for at least one hour. At the end of several hours, the child may be symptom free, and will remain symptom free until the next episode. While this is actually a migraine, there is typically no headache, which can make it difficult to diagnose. Once a physician has ruled out any problem related to the upper or lower gastrointestinal tract, and a physical examination reveals no signs of gastrointestinal disease, migraine syndrome should be considered. About one-fifth of these children experience actual headaches, and about one-third also have motion sickness, commonly car sickness. In fact, a large number of migraine patients have a history of car sickness as children, continuing into adulthood. In addition, there may be a history of allergies to inhalants. Although this syndrome can be seen in children from five to fifteen years of age, the average age of onset is just over five years old.

Abdominal migraine: While the children described above with severe vomiting don't always have abdominal pain, there is another migraine syndrome that involves recurrent abdominal pain. Children with abdominal migraines develop midline abdominal pain or pain around the umbilical area, which is usually described as dull or just sore, although it could be moderate to severe in intensity. These attacks of abdominal pain may last from one to 72 hours, and sometimes includes nausea and pallor of the face. Bear in mind that vomiting may not be associated with this abdominal pain disorder. In between attacks, the child feels completely normal. I have seen children who have experienced two hours of severe abdominal pain, but by the time they get to the office the pain is completely gone and the child is playing happily, as if nothing ever happened. This type of disorder can be labeled with different names, including irritable bowel syndrome, abdominal migraine, and dyspepsia. It is also associated with a higher risk of anxiety, headaches, and possible limb pain. Girls seem to develop abdominal migraine more than boys, and headaches are more likely to occur during this pain syndrome.

Benign paroxysmal vertigo of childhood: This condition is characterized by recurrent brief episodes of dizziness or vertigo occurring without warning and resolving spontaneously in otherwise healthy children. The attacks are not necessarily caused by a certain position or activity. They may occur at any time. Any type of dizziness or vertigo warrants a neurological examination, as well as hearing and vision testing. If these tests are normal, migraine may be the problem. In addition to the dizziness and vertigo, throbbing headaches may occur during these attacks. Children with this syndrome may also have some vomiting and rapid back-and-forth eye movements. Very young children, especially infants, may have a condition called benign paroxysmal torticollis, which involves recurrent episodes of head tilting to one side, perhaps with a slight rotation. These episodes will last minutes to days, and recur on a monthly basis. Along with these attacks the patient may have one or more of the following: pallor, irritability, malaise, vomiting or ataxia (loss of muscle coordination). There could be difficulty standing up and walking. Car sickness is by far the most common problem that I see in children suffering from this condition. They seem to outgrow these early symptoms, and develop migraine headaches as adults.

While each of these conditions can be very frightening for parents, they are benign problems, and all of them seem to respond to medication typically used for migraine patients, even though they may not have headaches associated with their condition. In fact, the headache is typically not the focus in children—it's the secondary symptoms that are more intense. If a head-ache does occur, children often experience migraine pain for a much shorter duration.

Keep in mind that while children may have different symptoms from adults, the migraine triggers are often the same. Dietary triggers, stress, lack of sleep, and other changes can produce a headache for a child who has a sensitive nervous system, just as with adults. Therefore, the same preventive measures outlined in this book for you can also be applied to your children. This can be especially difficult as children get older. We all know that teenagers like to stay up late and sleep until noon on the weekends. Also, many common dietary triggers, such as caffeine-laden soda and chocolate, are staples of the teenage diet. If your child is plagued by headaches, then keeping a diary, following a migraine diet, and enforcing good sleep habits can often provide relief without the use of medication.

CHAPTER 3

Ice Picks and Hot Dogs

You might be wondering what ice picks and hot dogs have to do with headaches. Well, they are just two of the many types or classifications of primary headaches. As I mentioned earlier, the International Headache Classification Subcommittee recognizes over 300 specific types of headaches—the majority of which are extremely rare. Over the years, the medical community has compiled massive amounts of headache research data in an attempt to better understand this complicated ailment. While we have come a long way in our ability to diagnose and treat headaches, there is still much to be learned.

To simplify, we can break down the list of primary headaches into four main classifications:

1. Migraine
2. Tension-type

3. Cluster (and its relatives)
4. Other—exertional, sexual, hormonal, etc.

Migraine is, by far, the most common headache treated by physicians, and there are some members of the medical community who believe nearly all primary headaches are really migraine; that is, they stem from the same mechanism as migraine and should be treated the same way. To muddy the waters further, some patients can have multiple diagnoses. They suffer from more than one distinct type of headache. For example, a patient may have migraine with aura, as well as frequent tension-type headaches. And finally, as we've discussed, headaches can change over time. What begins as a pattern of migraines with aura may evolve into chronic daily headaches without aura. Again, the complex and changeable nature of headaches make keeping a detailed headache diary critically important to finding a solution.

While it's impossible to describe every type of headache here, it might be helpful to look at some of the more common and interesting ailments. Headaches can be easily misinterpreted and misdiagnosed, so having as much information as possible goes a long way toward developing an effective treatment plan. As you read the following, you may find yourself nodding in recognition or saying "aha, that sounds like me."

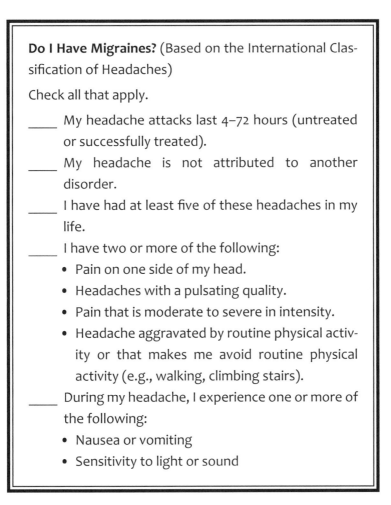

Do I Have Migraines? (Based on the International Classification of Headaches)

Check all that apply.

_____ My headache attacks last 4–72 hours (untreated or successfully treated).

_____ My headache is not attributed to another disorder.

_____ I have had at least five of these headaches in my life.

_____ I have two or more of the following:

- Pain on one side of my head.
- Headaches with a pulsating quality.
- Pain that is moderate to severe in intensity.
- Headache aggravated by routine physical activity or that makes me avoid routine physical activity (e.g., walking, climbing stairs).

_____ During my headache, I experience one or more of the following:

- Nausea or vomiting
- Sensitivity to light or sound

Tension-Type Headaches

According to research, about 40 percent of the population has experienced a tension-type headache, making it the most common headache complaint. However, because they are typically not disabling, tension-type headaches are usually not treated by a physician. They are characterized by generally mild or dull pain that feels more like a tight band or constriction around the head rather than throbbing, and they are not normally accompanied by sensitivity to light or sounds, or nausea. Therefore, tension-type headaches rarely interfere with a person's life enough to seek medical treatment. That's not to say they aren't aggravating!

Tension-type headaches come in two varieties: episodic and chronic. Episodic tension headaches can be infrequent (fewer than one day per month) or frequent (up to 14 days per month). Chronic tension-type headache is defined as a headache that occurs on 15 or more days per month for at least three consecutive months. When this happens, tension-type headaches can become disabling and require treatment. Over time, patients with chronic tension-type headaches may also experience migraine symptoms, such as nausea or sensitivity to light and sounds, which makes an accurate diagnosis more difficult.

Because tension-type headaches are not well understood, they are diagnosed by what they *are not*, rather than by what they are. Instead of pain that throbs and becomes worse with activity, such as occurs with a migraine, tension-type headache pain is a more diffuse, nondescript ache. There is a common misconception that tension-type headaches are caused by tension built up from the workplace, or "sleeping wrong" the night

Do I Have Tension-Type Headaches? (Based on the International Classification of Headaches)

Check all that apply.

_____ My headache involves at least two of the following:
- Bilateral pain (pain on both sides of the head or across the forehead).
- A pressing or tightening quality (non-pulsating).
- Pain that is mild or moderate in intensity.
- Pain that is not aggravated by routine physical activity.

_____ I have both of the following:
- No nausea or vomiting.
- No more than one of photophobia or phonophobia.

_____ I have had at least ten episodes occurring less than one day a month and less than 12 days a year (infrequent tension-type headache).

_____ I have had at least ten episodes occurring on more than one but fewer than 15 days a month for more than three months (frequent tension-type headache).

_____ My head and/or neck is tender when manually palpated.

_____ My headaches are not attributable to another disorder.

before, resulting in a stiff neck. Although tension-type headaches are often accompanied by sore muscles in the head and neck, and sometimes the shoulder, excessive muscle tension is *not* the cause, which is why medical experts refer to it as a tension-*type* headache. Unlike migraine, which typically becomes worse with physical activity, tension-type headaches tend to respond well to mild activity.

Most often, tension-type headache sufferers can find relief from OTC medications. However, if your symptoms are not alleviated through self-medication, or if they impair your ability to function, you may want to visit your primary care physician. Migraines often masquerade as tension-type headaches; so, by the time a patient reaches the physician's office, the tension-type headache sufferer may, in fact, be a migraineur. What started out as a tension-type headache has actually transformed into a migraine with one-sided, pounding pain, accompanied by sensitivity to sound and light, and perhaps nausea.

Tension-type headaches and migraines often occur in the same individual, and the patient can usually tell the difference between the two. Keep in mind, the underlying mechanism could be the same in both conditions, and it's sometimes difficult to distinguish one from the other. It's also interesting to note that some tension-type headaches respond well to migraine-specific medications.

Cluster Headache

Oddly enough, although more women than men get headaches, in general, the cluster headache occurs eight times more often in men than women. Cluster headaches are less common than migraines or tension-type headaches, but they are notable due to their severity. They are usually unilateral (on one side of the head) and occur behind or around the eye, the temple, and the upper jaw. The pain is intense, and is described as piercing or boring. If you experience a cluster headache, you may also exhibit—on the headache side—a red, irritated eye, nasal congestion, runny nose, facial sweating, swelling of the eyelid or face, watering or tearing of the eye, a droopy eyelid, or a constricted pupil. At least one of these symptoms must be present to establish a diagnosis.

The term "cluster" refers to the pattern or intervals in which these headaches occur. Cluster headaches may strike daily or several times a day for weeks to months at a time, and then disappear for months. They typically last between 15 to 90 minutes, and usually occur at the same time each day or night. I had a patient whose headache occurred so regularly that he could set his alarm clock for about five minutes before the headache began. Because cluster headaches can be excruciating, they often cause a person to pace around the room, pound the head, and seek different positions or motions to find comfort, even rocking back and forth. Then, without warning, the headache leaves as fast it came, only to return again several hours later.

Medical experts are not sure what causes cluster headaches, although there is some correlation between men who suffer from cluster headaches and those who are heavy smokers and drinkers. In addition, I often see an increase in cluster headaches during the change in

---

Do I Have Cluster Headaches? (Based on the International Classification of Headaches)

Check all that apply.

____ My headaches are severe and one-sided, causing pain behind or around the eye, the temple, and/or jaw.

____ The pain lasts 15–90 minutes.

____ The pain has a piercing, boring quality.

____ My headache is accompanied by more than one of the following:

- A red, irritated eye and/or watery eye.
- Nasal congestion.
- Swelling of the eyelid.
- Facial sweating.
- A drooping eyelid and/or constricted pupil.

____ I have had at least 20 of these intense headaches.

____ My headaches are not attributable to another disorder.

---

seasons, especially in the spring, in early summer around the longest day of the year, and in early winter near the shortest day of the year. I have no explanation for this phenomenon other than to offer my observation.

Cluster headaches can be managed successfully with medication, and anyone who experiences these should see his or her physician for treatment. It's important for sufferers of this type of headache to use medication to abort an acute attack, as well as preventive medication to decrease the frequency and severity.

"I thought I had a brain tumor."

Ann is a 43-year-old woman who suffered from severe headaches on one side of her head for several years. The headache was accompanied by redness of her left eye, nasal discharge and stuffiness on the left side, and swelling of her eyelid and face. Initially, she was treated for migraine, and while some migraine medications seemed to help, none completely alleviated her symptoms. Frustrated, and concerned that she might have a brain tumor, she saw several neurologists for a complete work-up. The good news was that they didn't find a tumor or other secondary condition, such as blood vessel disease. The bad news was that she still suffered from these debilitating headaches.

She was treated with medications used for chronic tension-type headaches, but still found no relief. By the time she reached my office, she was at the end of her rope. After a thorough examination, she was diagnosed with *hemicrania continua*, a relative of the cluster headache. This persistent unilateral headache is usually found in women, and acts like a cluster headache: it is one-sided without shifting and can be continuous; it is moderate in intensity with exacerbations of severe pain; and the patient may also have the facial and eye symptoms that go along with cluster headaches. However, this particular type of headache responds almost completely to a drug called Indomethacin (an NSAID drug), which migraine and cluster headaches do not.

One of the reasons that Ann's diagnosis is difficult is the fact that she also had nausea and severe vomiting—two symptoms I would not expect to see in *hemicrania continua*. On further investigation, I found she also had gastritis and inflammation of the stomach caused by previous medications. This is a perfect example of why it's important to treat the whole person and not just the headaches. After stabilizing her stomach distress, I treated her with Indomethacin, which put an end to her severe headaches within a few weeks. Though Ann still has occasional headaches, she has not experienced anything like the *hemicrania continua* she had before, and is functioning much better.

Ice Pick Headache

This is one of the most curious headaches. Yes, it's called an ice pick headache because it sometimes feels like someone is actually stabbing you in the head with an ice pick. It causes a severe, jabbing pain that may occur several times a week or several times a day. These headaches typically last a few seconds to several minutes and then resolve. Unlike cluster headaches, ice pick headaches are not associated with any changes in the pupil or redness of the eye. There is no sensitivity to light or sounds, or nausea with these headaches, although ice pick headaches are very common in patients who experience migraines. In fact, they occur in about 40 percent of migraine patients, and usually occur in the same area of the head where the migraine occurs.

Unfortunately, treatment when an ice pick headache actually occurs is impractical because of the brevity and repetition of attacks. The medication Indomethacin given prophylactically (preventively) provides complete or partial improvement in most cases. Some patients also find relief by taking 3 to 12 mg of melatonin daily and 400 mg of Gabapentin (a drug used to treat epilepsy and neuropathic pain) twice a day.

Sexual Headache

The sexual or coital headache is fairly common and can be particularly disturbing. This type of headache is precipitated by sexual activity, occurring just prior to or during orgasm. It usually starts as a dull headache on both sides of the head, and often causes pain in the neck or jaw area. As the patient becomes sexually aroused and progresses toward orgasm, the headache quickly worsens until it becomes excruciating. Those who have experienced this type of headache describe it as an "explosion." Some patients also get a lesser, dull headache after sexual relations. These are not as severe as the headache that occurs with orgasm, but may linger a few hours and then resolve.

These headaches are actually migraines, and you guessed it: the trigger is the chemical and physical changes that occur in the body during sex. Of course, no one is suggesting you avoid this "trigger," but as with all migraines, you can avoid other potential triggers to lessen the occurrence. If cutting out caffeine and limiting other dietary triggers does not help, migraine medications may be the answer. Indomethacin taken before sexual relations can help to reduce or eliminate these headaches. However, with this headache, ruling out a more serious disorder is the first order of business.

Hot Dogs and Ice Cream

We have discussed dietary triggers such as caffeine, red wine, and MSG and their effects on migraine. In that same category, there is a specific headache that most people are familiar with; it is sometimes called a "brain freeze." This headache is caused by ice cream and other icy cold treats. It really starts at the back of the upper part of the mouth, when the cold food or beverage stimulates nerves in that spot, and travels to the center of the brain. It can last a few seconds to several minutes, and then disappears. Some people find relief by pressing the tongue against the roof of their mouth. Interestingly, people who frequently get ice cream headaches usually have had migraines or will develop migraines in the future.

Another interesting food-related headache is the hot dog headache. The culprit is really the preservatives, particularly nitrates and nitrites, which are found in hot dogs and other processed meats such as bologna, sausage, pepperoni, and salami. In people who are sensitive to these preservatives, the headache comes on fairly quickly after eating. If this happens to you, the best solution is to avoid hot dogs and other processed meats, or look for packages that say they are nitrate and nitrite free.

"Sinus" Headache

In many cases, migraine gets confused with sinus headache. This is a result of the complicated anatomy we discussed earlier. Migraine sends pain signals along nerve branches in both the head and the face, including the area below the eyes but above the upper lip, and into the sinus cavities. In addition, migraine can cause sinus-type symptoms such as nasal congestion and swelling of the face due to the inflammation of blood vessels. Most "sinus headaches" that recur over time are actually migraine. True sinus headaches typically occur along with head colds, a sinus (bacterial) infection, or a structural problem within the sinus cavities.

Whether allergies cause headaches or not is unclear, although many patients seem to be sensitive to certain types of food or inhalants. Patients may also be sensitive to grasses, trees, weeds, molds and dust mites, and these sensitivities may precipitate a headache. The best way to be certain is to see an allergist for testing and then treat accordingly.

Many patients will also complain of headaches when the barometric pressure changes, particularly when it dips. A change in weather, such as an approaching storm or low pressure system, can trigger a headache. However, this is not a sinus headache, but rather a migraine that is triggered by weather changes.

"My 'sinus infections' were really migraines."

Joe called my office every two weeks, like clockwork, requesting antibiotics to clear his sinus infection and headache. He told me it takes almost three days to calm the headache down after he takes the antibiotics, and then he feels good until the next attack about ten to fourteen days later. That's a lot of sinus infections! What is really going on here?

Infections of the sinuses may occur about a week or two after a respiratory infection that causes sneezing, runny nose, postnasal drip, and nasal congestion. After about two weeks of this, the sinus cavity can become obstructed and cause pain, usually accompanied by fever and pus-like discharge from the nose. In these cases, it does take about two weeks of antibiotics to clear the infection. Most of my patients who actually have a sinus infection describe the pain as a pressure rather than a headache, and not a very serious one. But, let's get back to Joe …

He describes his "sinus headache" as pain across the forehead and down the back of his neck, which disappears after three days. His symptoms are the same as a person with an early migraine—frontal head pain, fatigue, difficulty sleeping, and nasal congestion. He is not having any yellowish or yellowish-green discharge, and more importantly, is not experiencing an early upper respiratory infection. The fact that antibiotics seem to help in "about three days" is suspicious, because migraines typically resolve in three days. Furthermore, having a sinus infection every two weeks, or 24 sinus infections a year, means he would have a cold or upper respiratory infection every day, all year round!

What is actually happening is that the migraine mechanism is causing swelling of the blood vessels and mucus membranes of the nose. The openings that drain the sinus cavities have become occluded or obstructed due to the inflammation. This can certainly cause pressure and headaches as the migraine mechanism progresses. Migraine-specific medications, such as triptans, can reverse the process, relieving the pressure and the headache.

Joe was also making the situation worse by using lots of decongestant nasal spray, which caused rebound congestion—the more spray he used, the more congested he became and the more spray he needed. The first step was to discontinue using the nasal spray, along with any other type of congestion relief medication. Next, Joe was placed on a migraine diet and practiced the other non-pharmacological strategies we've discussed—consistent sleep patterns, regular meals, and a walking program. Today, he is free of headaches.

Like most of my patients who see me for chronic sinus headaches, Joe had nothing of the sort.

"I was a human weather barometer."

Diane was better at predicting the weather than many meteorologists. Unfortunately, she paid the price in the form of a terrible headache. It seemed as though every time the barometric pressure changed, signaling a storm or rise in humidity, she would get a headache. And, because her headaches almost always involved nasal congestion and the feeling of pressure behind her eyes, she mistakenly attributed them to a "sinus problem." She described the pain as "feeling like my eyeballs were going to pop out of my head."

Diane is not alone. Many migraine sufferers are affected by weather changes, and many of these patients believe they are having a sinus headache due to nasal congestion. In fact, the nasal congestion is not causing the pain, but rather the headache is causing the nasal congestion.

Facial pain, congestion, and pressure are symptoms of the migraine. That's why OTC medications used to treat congestion aren't effective, or provide only temporary relief. Actually, migraine pain can travel down the nerve branch that affects the face and sinus cavities.

The weather is a major trigger for Diane, but it's not the only one. By keeping a diary of her headaches, she discovered other contributing factors. Her headaches were worse around her menstrual period, and often occurred after drinking red wine during an evening out. Obviously, none of us can change the weather, but we can control other migraine triggers, which may lessen the frequency and severity of headaches when the barometer dips. Through a combination of dietary changes and a preventive migraine medication, Diane was able to effectively manage her headaches—although she can no longer predict the weather!

Chronic Daily Headache

Thankfully, this condition occurs infrequently (2–3 percent of the headache population). When it does occur, it is very difficult to treat. It often involves medication overuse, and secondary conditions such as anxiety or depression. As you can imagine, chronic daily headaches often impair a person's ability to function at work or in social situations.

Several patterns of chronic daily headaches have been observed. Often, the underlying pattern can be defined as a transformation from an episodic migraine, tension-type, or cluster headache, to a chronic daily headache that comes and goes. A second type of chronic daily headache can be a persistent daily headache of new onset. Patients can pinpoint exactly when the headache started, for example, following a viral infection. Still, a third type may emanate from head trauma or degenerative joint disease of the spine; therefore, it is classified as a secondary headache.

"My headache never went away."

Bill came to see me with an interesting history. On July 28, 2010, at exactly 3:00 P.M., while reading, he developed a severe headache that never went away. He went to see his family physician and was also seen by several specialists who assured him that nothing serious was going on, and that the headache should resolve. But it did not. In fact, Bill has not had a headache-free day since.

When I asked him to describe the headache, he said it was in the back of his head and encompassed the upper portion of his neck, wrapping around his head like a horseshoe. At times, he develops sensitivity to light and sounds, as well as nausea. On a 10-point pain scale, Bill's headache may be anywhere between 3 and 10, no matter what he does. Routine physical activities do not seem to make his headache worse, but nothing seems to make it better either.

The official diagnosis is "daily persistent headache," since Bill had no precipitating factors or prior headache history. Although this is a rare disorder, many of these patients also have migraine features. After extensive investigation, the cause of Bill's headache is still unknown. We have excluded more serious disorders, which is some comfort. We have also tried several preventive medications. Bill actually improved with a combination of valproic acid and non-pharmalogical treatment for migraines, as well as trigger-point injections. In cases such as these, when medications typically used to treat migraines have varying results, it takes some trial and error to find an effective treatment.

And the List Goes On

As mentioned, it would be virtually impossible to list all the types of headaches or headache triggers (see the list of potential triggers in Chapter 2). Headaches can occur at *higher altitudes* or due to *time changes* as you travel, and the resulting *sleep disruptions*. I have seen chronic headaches caused by *carbon monoxide* escaping through a heating system for months before being discovered. *Dental problems* such as a cracked or diseased tooth can also cause a severe headache. Patients may come in complaining about pain that radiates along the jaw or in the sinuses, which we trace back to a tooth that requires a root canal. Similarly, *TMJ disorder* (temporomandibular joint pain) will cause pain in the sinus and jaw area, as well as a headache, and is usually accompanied by clicking, slipping, or locking of the jaw joints. TMJ is not really a diagnosis in itself, but part of the headache complex. For some people, particularly those who are overweight, *sleep apnea* can lead to chronic headaches.

In addition, there are many secondary headaches that occur in certain populations. For instance, elderly patients can develop a specific headache that should be looked for and treated quickly—*giant cell arteritis,* which affects the temporal arteries in the head. Inflammation of the artery occurs, and the blood vessel may become clogged or compromised due to this inflammation. One of the symptoms we look for in this diagnosis is claudication (discomfort or pain) of the jaw while chewing. The patient will also have tenderness over the temporal artery. If this condition is suspected, it's important to test and treat quickly because non-treatment may cause permanent blindness.

Again, there are many diseases and medical conditions that can cause secondary headaches—conditions which go beyond the scope of this book. Any headache that is new, suddenly severe, or is accompanied by new-onset seizures warrants a visit to your primary care physician. No one knows your body as well as you. Therefore, as with all medical conditions, you are the best judge of what changes seem abnormal or when you feel something is "just not right." Don't hesitate to follow your intuition.

"Can running cause a blood vessel to burst?"

Jack was in excellent physical condition. He was a long-distance runner who competed on his college track team. Then one day, he started to get headaches near the end of his run that would last a couple of hours. He started taking some OTC medications, which seemed to help initially, but over time, the headaches became worse.

However, he did not seek treatment until he experienced something that frightened him. Following a 10K race, Jack was struck with an intense, one-sided headache, accompanied by severe vomiting, and sensitivity to light and sound. The headache lasted several hours and then resolved. He was concerned that he had burst a blood vessel in his brain while running.

Certainly, a headache like this should be taken seriously, because it could indeed indicate a hemorrhage or burst blood vessel. Luckily, after a complete evaluation of his tests, which were negative, he was diagnosed with an *exertional headache.* Many patients, like Jack, who suffer from *exertional headaches,* will also have a history of migraine or other type of headache—but they should never be taken lightly.

Exercise-induced headaches can be exacerbated by factors such as high temperatures and humidity, high altitudes, hypoglycemia, and caffeine. Medication is not always needed when treating exertional headaches. Many patients benefit from simple preventive measures, such as warming up prior to exercising, eating properly, and avoiding caffeine. When these strategies aren't enough, taking Indomethacin or Naprosyn before exercising may be helpful. Beta-adrenergic blockers may also be prescribed for three to six months, after which the disorder typically resolves.

Headaches in Women

When it comes to women and headaches, hormones are a notorious trigger. Headaches affect women differently throughout their life stages.

Menstrual Periods: *About 70 percent of migraine sufferers are female and about 70 percent of those female migraine sufferers describe a relationship between their headaches and their menstrual periods. Menstrual migraines have been defined as acute migraine attacks that occur days before the menstrual period, or 2–3 days into menstruation. Some women may also have migraines at other times of the month, as well as menstrual migraines. However, according to these women, the menstrual migraines are greater in length, intensity, and severity. They may also have more premenstrual headaches. Headaches that occur before the menstrual cycle are categorized as migraine, tension-type, or a combination of both. These headaches are part of a whole range of symptomatology commonly called premenstrual syndrome (PMS), which can affect women physically, psychologically, and emotionally. Associated complaints may include fatigue, food cravings, fluid retention, joint* pain, breast tenderness, anxiety, depression, impaired memory, irritability, and paranoia.

The hormones that trigger menstrual migraines, as well as the symptoms listed above, are estrogen and progesterone—the levels of these hormones seem to affect the severity and duration of these headaches. Many of these women have such severe headaches they must take time off from work and are not able to function normally for several days. This pattern is fairly consistent from month to month. Both abortive and preventive migraine medications can be used to manage menstrual migraines.

Migraine attacks are also associated with dysmenorrhea—very painful periods. In this case, menstrual migraines are often treated with a non-steroidal anti-inflammatory drug (NSAID), such as ibuprofen or naproxen sodium. Steady use of these medications starting three days prior to the start of the menstrual period and continued through the period is helpful in decreasing both the frequency and severity of migraine attacks. With the use of an NSAID, migraine-specific medication such as a triptan may be more effective.

Pregnancy: For many women who suffer from menstrual migraines—about 70 percent—their headaches improve or disappear during pregnancy. This is probably due to the high, steady level of estrogen produced during this time. Headaches may persist during the first trimester of pregnancy, and then decrease markedly or even resolve completely during the second and third trimesters. Unfortunately, headaches seem to reappear during the postpartum period and eventually escalate to the same level of intensity as were experienced before pregnancy.

Migraines occurring postpartum are related to the drop in estrogen and progesterone following delivery. These patients should also watch for postpartum depression, which may be more serious in headache-prone women. Breast-feeding is believed to provide some protection against migraine attacks. Again, this is probably associated with the change in estrogen and progesterone levels, and perhaps the decreased number of periods during this time. There is probably little change in migraine frequency during lactation.

Menopause: This life stage seems to affect women differently. For most women, the fluctuation of estrogen levels may gradually decrease migraine headaches, and often lessen the severity of those attacks. The headaches may even cease altogether. However, some women find their headaches become worse during this time, and others actually experience the onset of migraines during menopause. Interestingly, those patients who experience a decrease in migraines during menopause may have an increase in tension headaches.

Because the majority of female migraine sufferers find relief from migraines during menopause, it has been advocated by some women to have a hysterectomy or ovary removal (i.e., surgical menopause) to "cure" migraines. This is a drastic treatment without a guarantee. Studies have found that in some patients who have undergone such surgeries, headaches are unchanged or made worse. Therefore, I would not advise any surgical procedure to remove the uterus or ovaries in order to decrease the frequency or intensity of migraine headaches.

Hormone Replacement Therapy: Hormonal Replacement Therapy (HRT) is a combination of estrogen and progesterone in low doses. The low dosage may be helpful to some migraine patients. However, in many cases, no matter the hormone levels administered, HRT can exacerbate migraines that would otherwise decrease or resolve after menopause. In addition, HRT can cause other side effects, which may militate against their use. Often it is a matter of trial and error in finding the type and dosage that works best for an individual, if HRT is warranted.

Oral Contraceptives: Oral contraceptives can be a two-edged sword. The stabilization of estrogen and progesterone can be a factor in stabilizing headaches; however, in most cases, birth control pills can actually exacerbate migraines. Patients who have migraines with aura are also at a greater risk for stroke while taking oral contraceptives, especially if they are over 35 years old and smoke.

Triphasic or biphasic birth control pills are so named because there is a gradual escalation of hormonal content. In most of the birth control pill packages, the last seven days consist of a placebo—pills without any estrogen or progesterone, which in essence causes the period. The migraine patient is more vulnerable to headaches with these combinations than if taking those pills that have the same estrogen or progesterone content for the full 20–21 days. If oral contraceptives are necessary, there is a way of using smaller doses of estrogen or introducing small amounts of estrogen during the placebo period, which may decrease headaches. Another option is to use birth control pills continuously for three consecutive months and not use the placebo portion, allowing the patient to have a menstrual period every three months. This can stabilize the headaches and allow the physician some time to add in both acute and preventive migraine medications.

(For more information about migraine medications, as well as alternate delivery systems for severe headaches or patients with a tendency toward nausea and vomiting, please refer to Chapter 5.)

Headaches in Seniors

They say growing old is not for sissies, and I would agree. There are many health concerns that are unique to seniors. When it comes to headaches, any headache that begins in patients older than 50 is always suspicious. It could be related to organic problems such as brain tumors, strokes, diseases of the blood vessels in the head, among other problems. One diagnosis not to miss is giant cell temporal arteritis.

Giant cell temporal arteritis occurs when the temporal artery located in the temple at the side of the head becomes inflamed and causes a localized headache. When it is touched, there is usually tenderness over the temporal artery on one side of the head. Lab tests including sed rate (a blood test that can reveal inflammatory activity in your body) along with a temporal artery biopsy will confirm the diagnosis. The headache, if left untreated, can lead to blindness, which is why it's very important to diagnose this condition early. Once diagnosed, it can be alleviated with high-dose steroids taken for several weeks and then gradually tapering them off.

The second type of headache to watch for in seniors is the hypnic headache, which occurs 15 times per month or more. Strangely enough, it happens only during sleep and wakes the patient up. Patients who have this type of headache do not experience photophobia, phonophobia, or nausea. They describe the pain as dull, but enough to rouse them from sleep, even during a nap. Successful treatment involves bedtime doses of lithium carbonate (300–600 mg).

A third type of headache seen in seniors is called trigeminal neuralgia, which consists of sudden, violent bursts of stabbing pain lasting from a fraction of a second to many minutes. These headaches can affect the second trigeminal nerve over the face between the nose and the ear, or the third trigeminal nerve over the jaw area. Treatment usually consists of the medications Baclofen, Carbamazepine, or Gabapentin. In extreme cases, when medication is ineffective, surgery can be performed using a microvascular decompression procedure.

Thankfully, most headaches in seniors do not fall into these categories. Like most migraines, they are usually related to food or drink. Take Greg for example: Greg is a 75-year-old man who came to see me with dull, diffuse headaches which occurred daily. Occasionally, he had a loss of vision in his left eye for 20 minutes at a time, and then became asymptomatic. Though his tests were negative, his cardiologist still felt this indicated a blood clot problem and gave him blood thinners, which did not seem to help. Several months prior to visiting his cardiologist, Greg's primary care physician recommended that he drink a couple of glasses of red wine each night to help reduce his cholesterol and ease his anxieties. He had been very concerned about a child in his family who was having some health problems. After reviewing his lab tests, x-rays, and general medical history, I found nothing to suggest a blood clot or other health issue. I asked him to discontinue the red wine, and to make certain he ate three meals a day, along with some healthy snacks between meals if he was hungry. Within a short time, both his headaches and eye problems resolved very nicely.

CHAPTER *4*

Taking Control—Part I

Whatever form your headaches take, from episodic severe migraines to chronic daily pain, the good news is that you don't have to continue to suffer. You can take control of the situation and eliminate, or dramatically reduce, your headaches. Of course, headache management is not always easy, and it often requires time and commitment to certain lifestyle changes. I understand that's easier said than done. When you're in pain, it's natural to want a quick fix—*just give me a pill and make it go away!* Yes, there are many highly effective medications available for the prevention and relief of migraines, and we will discuss those options in the next chapter; however, the best treatment plans consist of both the proper use of medication *and* lifestyle modifications.

This is true with many medical conditions. Just as cholesterol-reducing medication is more effective when combined with appropriate diet and exercise, migraine medications are better able to do their job when patients understand the reasons for their headaches, and take steps to alleviate them. In addition, many medications, when used too frequently or improperly, can make your condition worse by causing rebound headaches (see Chapter 5). While some headache sufferers find that with certain lifestyle changes they are able to avoid medication altogether, most often it is a combination of the two that ultimately provides long-term relief. That's why I want to start with a discussion of non-pharmacological headache management and the important role it plays in knocking out headaches.

Keeping a Headache Diary

As mentioned earlier, the first step in treating your headaches is to understand them. By keeping a thorough diary of your headaches, you and your physician will be able to identify triggers and recognize patterns, which will lead to a more successful treatment plan, and later help you fine-tune an existing regimen. I know what you're saying: *I already have enough to do in my daily life without adding another task.* That may be true, but consider the time you spend keeping a headache diary an investment in your health and well-being. If headaches are disrupting your life, can you afford *not* to take the necessary steps to get rid of them?

It's important to be very accurate when keeping a headache diary. Over time, the diary will reveal important clues, such as timing—when the headaches begin, what part of the day, day of the week, or week of the month they are more prevalent. It will also record the duration and severity of your headaches. Use a scale of 0 to 10 to indicate the level of pain you experience: 0 being no headache, and 10 being the most severe headache you've ever had. When I ask patients to describe headache pain, I use these general guidelines: severe headaches keep you home from work and in bed; moderate headaches allow you to stick it out, but you are suffering quite a bit; and mild headaches are noticeable but do not interfere with your tasks.

When keeping a diary, you should:

- Record the date and time the headache began.
- Indicate the intensity of the pain, using the 0 to 10 scale, as well as what part of the head is affected, including your neck and shoulders.
- Notice what you were doing when the headache began—exercising, working, resting, or reading, for example.
- List any associated symptoms, such as phonophobia (sensitivity to sound), photophobia (sensitivity to light), nausea, or vomiting.

- Note what you ate or drank in the 24-hour period prior to the onset of your headache, particularly known dietary migraine triggers.
- Jot down how you were feeling before the headache occurred—were you angry, sad, stressed out, or feeling depressed?
- Explain what you did to make yourself feel better, such as resting in a dark room, or taking OTC painkillers or migraine medications. Did these help? Did anything make you feel worse—physical activity, bright lights, or loud noises?
- For women, note whether you are on your menstrual period or what day of the cycle you are on.
- Record when the headache subsided.

For a sample headache diary, see Appendix I in the back of the book. Be sure to put your headache diary somewhere handy and noticeable, such as the refrigerator or next to your bed, so you don't forget to use it. Fill out the diary for at least a month before you bring it to your physician.

It may seem like a lot of information, especially if you are experiencing a headache, but the more thorough and accurate your diary is, the clearer the picture becomes. Sometimes, certain patterns or triggers are readily apparent, and other times, it may take months. Be patient and hang in there.

Lifestyle Changes

If you think of the migraine as a battleground on which you are continually up against the forces that cause your headaches, you begin to understand how the choices you make on a daily basis can affect the outcome. Asking someone to change his or her lifestyle can seem overwhelming at first, but keep in mind that even small changes can have a big impact. In addition, some of the same lifestyle changes that reduce the frequency and severity of headaches also provide other health benefits, such as less stress, more energy, and weight loss.

When it comes to lifestyle, the key aspects of headache management are sleep, exercise, posture/body alignment, and diet.

Sleep

Let's face it: most people don't get enough sleep. In fact, the Center for Disease Control and Prevention (CDC) estimates that 50 to 70 million Americans have some type of sleep or wakefulness disorder. Lack of sleep is increasingly linked to motor vehicle crashes and occupational accidents. People with sleep inefficiency are also more likely to suffer from chronic diseases, such as hypertension, diabetes, depression, obesity, and—you guessed it—migraines.

In fact, many of my patients with migraine do not sleep well. They either have trouble getting to sleep or have difficulty staying asleep. Many describe their sleep as "restless." One of the best things you can do to ensure you are getting proper rest and stave off headaches is to regulate your sleep patterns. Try to go to sleep at the same time every night, and wake up at the same time every morning. No exceptions—even on the weekends when you might want to sleep in. Set your alarm for the time you normally wake up. If you're feeling really tired try getting up and having something to eat, and then returning to bed for a little while longer. Just keep in mind that too much sleep can trigger a headache, just like too little shuteye.

You can also make your bedroom more restful by keeping it dark and cool, and banishing all electronics from your bedtime routine. Avoid caffeine and other stimulants late in the day, and find a relaxing bedtime ritual that works for you. There are many books and websites that offer tips and techniques for getting a good night's sleep. Suffice it to say, proper sleep is key to managing migraines. Not only are disrupted sleep patterns a known migraine trigger, but lack of sleep also makes it more difficult to cope with daily demands, which leads to more stress—and that leads to more headaches. If all non-pharmalogical methods fail to work and a patient is really struggling with sleep, a small dose (5–10 mg) of a tricyclic antidepressant, such as Amitriptyline, may help normalize a sleep pattern.

Sleep apnea is also a common cause of migraines, especially in individuals who are overweight. It's characterized by abnormal pauses in breathing or very shallow breathing during sleep. If you suspect that you have a sleep disorder, or have been diagnosed with sleep apnea, discuss the headache connection with your physician.

Exercise

Over the years, I have found that many migraine patients lack physical activity and general fitness. Interestingly, the reasons they give for not exercising—not enough time for themselves, too much work, too many obligations, and no energy—are the very reasons they should be exercising! Most migraine patients would rather sit and relax when they have spare time, particularly after a migraine attack. But, it's important to get up and start moving. Even moderate exercise can help reduce stress and increase energy. A simple walking routine of 20–30 minutes per day, at least four days a week, can have a significant impact on your health and improve your quality of life. If you've been very inactive, try starting off by taking a five-minute walk outside each day and building from there. Of course, you should consult your physician about what's right for your particular health situation before beginning any exercise plan.

While you're thinking about exercise, let me say a word about your feet. You might not think your feet have anything to do with headache pain, but they can. If you are a runner or regular walker, make certain your shoes have good arch support and a wide toe box that gives your toes plenty of room. Also, be sure to replace your shoes when they get worn. I have seen time and again patients coming in with athletic shoes that are completely broken down and offering little support. Ideally, athletic shoes should be replaced every 200–300 miles, even if they look fine on the outside, because the internal structure weakens. When you are pounding the pavement, there is a tremendous amount of vibration as your feet hit the ground, and this vibration travels up the spine and into the neck and head. Constant pounding with improper shoes can stimulate those trigger points that cause headaches.

In addition to a regular fitness routine, specific neck exercises can be very beneficial to headache patients. Because the trigger points in the neck are stimulatory to headaches, doing exercises to improve range of motion and reduce stiffness are important. I often prescribe a series of basic neck exercises to headache patients to be done twice a day, every day. Heat can also be applied to the neck and shoulders to loosen stiff muscles, in conjunction with these exercises.

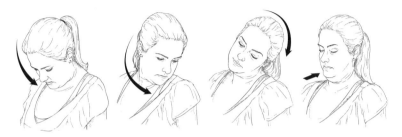

Exercise 1: Bend your chin to your chest and then rotate your chin to each shoulder. Tip your head toward each shoulder. Finally, pull in your chin make a double chin.

Exercise 2: Sit or stand up straight and raise shoulders up. Lower them back down and relax. Raise shoulders up again, and push them back. Lower and relax. Raise shoulders up again, and push them forward. Lower and relax.

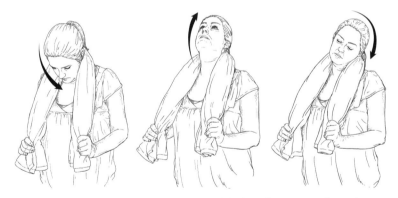

Exercise 3: Hold a rolled up towel behind your neck and gently pull down. Tilt chin down to chest. Tilt chin up toward ceiling. Tilt ears back and forth to each shoulder.

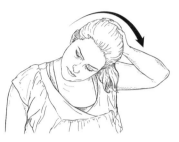

Exercise 4: Tilt your ear to your shoulder on the same side, and then tilt your chin forward and toward the opposite breast. Press with your hand gently to increase the stretch.

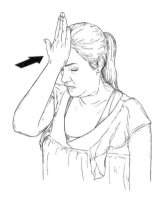

Exercise 5: Place palm on forehead and press head against palm, keeping your hand stationary and creating resistance between palm and head. Repeat on each side of head.

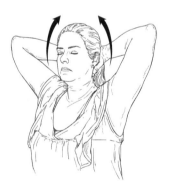

Exercise 6: Interlace fingers and place behind your neck at the base of your head. Pull elbows forward and up to create the sensation of lifting your head up and out of neck.

Exercise 7: Look straight ahead. Push chin forward away from neck creating a "turtle" effect. With head forward, turn neck side-to-side and up slightly.

Adapted from *The Woman's Migraine Toolkit,* Marcus, Dawn, and Bain, Philip, DiaMedica 2010

Stretching exercises which target muscles in the neck and shoulder area may be used to help reduce headache frequency and severity. During a mild headache, or as a headache begins, stretching can also help reduce the pain and prevent the headache from worsening. If you have significant neck pain or muscle tightness, you may want to consider seeing a physical therapist for an evaluation and treatment.

Did you know?

Studies suggest that four out of five people with headaches have problems with neck posture, and tender muscles in the head, neck, and shoulders that may be aggravating their headaches. In fact, many headache sufferers are also diagnosed with *myofascial pain syndrome*, which means the muscles become very tight and tender, and may cause shooting pain when pressed. Physical therapy, aerobic exercise, or stretching exercises such as yoga, Pilates, or Tai Chi can help reduce excessive muscle tension, and in turn, alleviate headaches.

Since muscle spasm can also trigger migraines, it makes sense that exercising to condition muscles can help reduce headaches. Exercise in general can play an important role in headache relief. In one study, headache sufferers who did aerobic exercise three times per week for six weeks experienced a nearly 45 percent reduction in headache severity.

Posture/Body Alignment

It's amazing to me how many people have poor posture. To see if your posture is correct, try placing a book on your head and balancing it as you walk around the house, or set a tissue box on your head while you work on the computer or read a book. It's not as easy as it looks! Playing the piano is also an excellent exercise for improving posture. Pianists are taught to adjust their seats and heads properly in order to view the music and play the keys without slouching, which is why they can play for several hours without fatigue. The fact is, slouching and improper head/neck alignment (i.e., the head is thrust forward) puts unhealthy pressure on the spine and neck, setting off those trigger points and causing headaches.

Ergonomics is the study of designing equipment and devices that fit the human body and its movements, thereby reducing strain on your back, shoulders, and neck. If you work at a computer all day, it may be worth your while to have someone who specializes in ergonomics come to your work station and assess the placement of your chair, keyboard, and other equipment, and make any necessary adjustments. It's also important to get up and take frequent breaks during the day to avoid eye strain and alleviate the tension in your neck and shoulders—perhaps doing the neck exercises we discussed earlier.

At home, one of the worst things you can do is to use your laptop or read in bed, which does not provide proper back and neck support. This slouching posture can cause muscle fatigue and even spasm. Carrying heavy backpacks or overloaded briefcases alters your posture as you lift and walk. Sometimes small adjustments in the way you do everyday tasks can not only prevent headaches, but save you grief in the future by avoiding structural problems in your back, shoulders, and neck.

Diet

As noted in Chapter 2, dietary triggers are the most common culprit in migraines. Reducing your exposure to certain foods and beverages can significantly decrease the occurrence of headaches. We have also learned that migraine triggers are cumulative, so the more of them you can decrease, the better you will feel. And yet, this is the area where I find that patients may be the most resistant. Nobody wants to give up their favorite foods or beverages—and many tell me they cannot live without caffeine!

The cumulative and fluctuating effect of dietary triggers can also be tricky. You might be able to have a glass of wine or a piece of chocolate on any given day without negative side effects. There may be a delay of a day, or even a number of days, from the time the food is consumed, until the time a headache begins. And remember our glass-of-water analogy: if enough triggers are added to your glass, it will spill over and cause a headache. So, that wine and chocolate that posed no problem on a day when you had a good night's sleep and it was clear and sunny outside can have an entirely different effect on a day when you are sleep deprived or rain is in the forecast. Keep an eye on your glass—are your triggers accumulating and making it full?

Do you find it hard to live without your afternoon caffeine fix? Well, if you suffer from migraines, you are consorting with the enemy! Caffeine produces a paradoxical effect that, in the beginning, may be helpful with headaches for a short period of time. In fact, some OTC painkillers contain caffeine to make them more effective. However, in the long run, caffeine will make the situation worse. It has a rebound effect, requiring the patient to consume more and more caffeine, and then withdrawal actually causes headaches to increase.

Over the years, the medical community has identified a list of common dietary migraine triggers, which includes alcohol (particularly red wine and champagne), chocolate, caffeine, aged cheeses, monosodium glutamate (MSG), aspartame (NutraSweet), nuts, and nitrates. This list is by no means all-inclusive. There may be certain foods or beverages that are unique triggers to you, which is why the migraine diary is so helpful. **The only way to know whether a certain food or beverage**

**is a trigger is to eliminate it completely from your diet
and see what happens.** I typically have patients remove
all potential triggers from their diet, and eventually add
them back in, one at a time, to pinpoint their particular
offenders. As a general rule, do not begin adding foods
or beverages back into your diet for two to three months,
and then be sure to only **add one item at a time.** This is
the only way to determine whether that particular food
or beverage is a trigger for you. However, there are certain items that should *never* be reintroduced into your
diet if you are headache prone. I'm sure you can guess
what they are: caffeine, MSG, artificial sweeteners, and
chocolate. Sorry.

"I had supersized headaches."

Dan developed what he described as "killer headaches"
when he was in his forties. He started having them once in
a while and eventually developed a headache every two
to three days, which is when he decided to seek treatment. A physical exam and routine tests showed that he
was in good health, so we began to look at some lifestyle
issues. My first question was "how many cups of coffee
do you drink each day?" What I should have asked was
"how big are the cups?"

We live in a "supersized" society. Coffee and soda are
no longer served in reasonable portions—they come in
giant, mega-sized jugs! A real cup is eight ounces, not
24, 48, or even 64-ounces, which is what people typically

order. In addition, many people have developed a habit of filling a huge container with soda and then sipping it through a straw all day long at their desks, which makes it difficult to keep track of how much you are actually drinking. If it's sitting there, it's also too tempting. I always advise patients to get rid of the container on their desk. When you're thirsty, get up and grab a bottle of water instead. And, when your doctor asks you how many cups of coffee, tea, or soda you consume, be sure to provide an accurate amount!

In Dan's case, not only was he drinking several "grande" coffees, at 16 ounces each, he was also downing an extra-large diet soda every afternoon at his desk. The combination of caffeine and artificial sweeteners were definite headache triggers for him, which was probably aggravated by sitting in front of a computer for eight to ten hours each day at work. Once he switched to decaf, replaced the soda with water, and made some ergonomic corrections to his workspace, his headaches went away.

Based on this list of common culprits, we have outlined a sample migraine diet. In general, the migraine diet limits tyramine, which is produced in foods from the natural breakdown of the amino acid tyrosine. Tyramine is not added to foods, but its levels increase in foods when they are aged, fermented, stored for long periods of time, or not fresh. The diet also avoids caffeine, alcohol, and MSG.

Eating to Prevent Migraine

Foods you can eat safely	Foods to avoid
Beverages:	
Decaffeinated coffee, natural fruit juice, club soda, non-cola soda (e.g., lemon-lime and ginger ale), non-alcoholic beer substitutes.	Chocolate, cocoa, and alcoholic beverages, particularly red wine and champagne. Caffeinated coffee, tea, or cola.
Bread and cereal:	
Commercial breads such as white, whole wheat, rye, French, Italian, English muffins, melba toast, crackers and bagels. All hot and cold cereals, including oatmeal, cornflakes, or bran cereal.	Fresh, homemade yeast bread; bread or crackers containing cheese; fresh yeast coffee cake, doughnuts, sourdough bread, and products that contain chocolate or nuts.
Dairy products:	
Milk: whole, 2% or skim. Cheese: cottage, cream, farmer, ricotta or processed. Limit yogurt to ½ cup per day.	Cultured dairy products, such as buttermilk and sour cream; chocolate milk. Cheese: bleu, boursault, brick, camembert, cheddar, Swiss (Emmentaler), Gouda, Roquefort, Stilton, mozzarella, parmesan, provolone, romano. (The more aged, the worse.)

Fruit:

All, except the few listed at right, unless your physician tells you otherwise.
Limit citrus fruit to ½ cup per day.

Avocados, bananas, cherries, figs, raisins, dried fruit, papaya, fruit cocktail, passion fruit, and red plums.

Meat, fish poultry:

Fresh or frozen turkey, chicken, fish, beef, lamb, veal, pork, tuna and tuna salad.
Limit eggs to three a week.

Aged, canned, cured, smoked or processed meat; canned or aged ham; pickled herring; salted and dried fish; chicken liver; aged game; hot dogs, bologna; fermented sausage (salami or pepperoni), bacon; meat prepared with a meat tenderizer; soy sauce or yeast extract; all foods with nitrites, nitrates, or amines.

Potato, rice, or pasta:

White, red, or sweet potatoes; rice and all pasta.

None.

Soup:

Cream soups made from allowable foods; homemade broth.

Canned soup, bouillon cubes, soup base with yeast or monosodium glutamate (read labels).

Vegetables and legumes:

All except those listed at right, unless your physician specifically tells you otherwise.

Pole or broad beans, lima or Italian beans, lentils, snow peas, fava beans, navy beans, pinto beans, pea pods, sauerkraut, garbanzo beans, onions (except for flavoring), olives, and pickles.

Sweets and dessert:

Sugar, jelly, jam, honey, hard candy.

Cocoa, chocolate candy or syrup.

Fruit allowed in diet, ice milk, cake and cookies made without chocolate or yeast; gelatin.

Mincemeat pie, ice cream, pudding, cookies or cake containing chocolate.

Miscellaneous:

Salt, in moderation; natural lemon juice, butter or margarine, cooking oil, whipped cream, white vinegar, and commercial salad dressing in small amounts.

Cheese sauce; soy sauce; monosodium glutamate (MSG); yeast; yeast abstract; brewer's yeast; meat tenderizer; and seasoned salt. Mixed dishes, such as macaroni and cheese, beef stroganoff, cheese blintzes, frozen dinners, pizza and lasagna. All nuts and seeds, including peanut butter. Oriental foods prepared with MSG. Any pickled, preserved or marinated foods. Some snack items (read labels).

How to Cheat

So, you've been following the migraine diet, but find yourself in a situation where following it seems impossible. Perhaps you've been invited to a dinner party where the hostess has gone all out, including presenting a lovingly prepared chocolate torte—how can you disappoint her and say no? Or, maybe you're out with friends and would like to join in the festivities by ordering just one drink without suffering from a headache later. There are times and ways to "cheat" a bit on your diet. Here are a few suggestions:

Shaken, not stirred—James Bond may have the right idea when it comes to alcohol and migraine prevention. If you have an alcoholic beverage, try ordering vodka, which seems to be well tolerated by headache sufferers. The better the quality of the vodka, the better it will be tolerated. And don't mix it with sugary juices or soft drinks—straight is best. In between sips, be sure to drink plenty of water. Of course, all alcohol should be consumed in moderation, especially if you are prone to headaches.

Make a choice. Go ahead and have a slice of that tempting chocolate torte, but try to make it small. And, realize that you are trying to keep your glass from overflowing; so if you choose to indulge in the chocolate dessert, you need to pass on other dietary triggers. Skip the glass of red wine with dinner or the cured meats and olives served beforehand.

Many patients will say "Hey, it's my anniversary, and I'm going to have a glass of wine," or something to that *effect. And, I always say, "That's fine, as long as you under-stand the possible consequences." It's okay to cheat once in a while, but if you get a headache, don't assume you need a new medication or a stronger pill. Do the best you can, deal with the results of your choices, and then make the next day better.*

Some rules of thumb for following your migraine prevention diet:

- Do not skip meals—fluctuations in blood sugar can cause headaches.
- Have three or more small meals a day.
- Eat at the same times each day.
- Eat all foods in moderation.
- Do not fast.

Migraine patients must eat on time. Skipping meals or eating on an erratic schedule will only aggravate your headaches. Many of my patients (about 50 percent) say they don't eat breakfast. I think it's very important to start the day with a meal, even if it's small. Some head-ache sufferers feel nauseated in the mornings. If that's you, try eating a few small tablespoons or bites of food, such as cereal, oatmeal or a granola bar, and then build from there. Most people find that the nausea slowly subsides once you get something in your stomach. Also, some patients tell me they get fatigued between meals, which can be due to a vacillation of blood sugar. Hypoglycemia, or low blood sugar, can certainly trigger headaches. But, don't reach for a piece of candy or other sugary treat to correct the situation. This will increase your blood sugar, but it will drop again quickly. What you need are complex carbohydrates, such as fresh fruit. Eating an apple, a pear, an apricot, a peach, or grapes will stabilize blood sugar without the crash.

A Note About Weight Loss

Some patients experience the added benefit of weight loss while on the migraine prevention diet, which is great. However, if one of your goals is to lose weight, be very careful in your plan. Diet pills and supplements that suppress your appetite or increase metabolism are migraine triggers. In addition, protein drinks, energy bars, and "light" frozen dinners may be high in MSG, and likely to blow your head off! Look for hidden sources of both caffeine and MSG by carefully reading nutritional labels.

Headache-Proofing Your Home

There are some simple changes you can make around your home that can help reduce headaches, and help you better cope with them when they occur. For instance, fluorescent lighting should be avoided, because bright lights are a headache trigger. Softer, incandescent lights which are designed for reading are a better choice. Chandeliers with multiple lights can also be jarring. If possible, install dimmer switches on overhead lights, so the brightness can be controlled. I often suggest "quiet areas" for my patients, which could be a den or other out-of-the-way room, where the door can be closed. Install a comfortable chair in this haven, which can be used for rest and relaxation. You can even put a sign on the door such as "Mommy is resting," to signal to the rest of the family this is your quiet time.

Sometimes, all it takes is 30 minutes of rest and quiet to stave off a headache. Of course, there should be no television, cell phones, computers or other disrupting

---

Let's Review:

- Begin keeping an accurate headache diary that will help you and your physician identify patterns and triggers.

- Make healthy lifestyle changes to prevent headaches and make any migraine medications more effective. Lifestyle changes may include: regular sleep habits, moderate exercise, good posture/body alignment and eliminating known dietary triggers.

- Headache-proof your home with softer lights and a quiet area where you can rest and relax without interruptions.

Ten Simple Things You Can Do to Reduce Stress and Promote Happiness

1. Try writing your thoughts and feelings down in a journal (or even on a piece of paper you can throw away), which can help you clarify things and give you a new perspective.

2. Do something you enjoy every day—and then do something for someone else.

3. When the stress of having to get a job done gets in the way of getting the job done, try a diversion—a voluntary change in activity or environment. It may be just what you need.

4. Talk it out. Discuss your problems and concerns with a trusted friend, which can help you clear your mind and see solutions more readily.

5. Accept the fact that we live in an imperfect world, and adopt a forgiving view of events and people.

6. Learn to delegate responsibilities to others who are capable.

7. Forget multitasking and do one thing at a time. When you are with someone, be with that person fully. When you are busy with a project, concentrate on doing that project and forget about everything else you have to do.

8. Inoculate yourself against a feared event. For example, before speaking in public, take time to go over every part of the experience in your mind. Imagine what you'll wear, what the audience will look like, how you will present your talk, etc. Visualize the

> *experience the way you want it to be. By the time the event arrives, you may find that it will be "old hat" and much of your anxiety has vanished.*
>
> 9. *Schedule a realistic day. Avoid the tendency to schedule back-to-back appointments, allowing time to breathe in between.*
>
> 10. *Adopt an optimistic view of the world. Believe that most people are doing the best they can, including yourself, and eliminate negative or destructive self-talk: "I'm too old to ... " or "I'm too out-of-shape for ... "*

electronics in this room, although soft, soothing music is advisable. If you are unable to claim a room for yourself, you might try a warm, relaxing bath. This would also give you a chance to loosen tight muscles and practice those range of motion exercises on your neck. While candles may seem like a soothing addition to your relaxation time, be wary. Scented candles can aggravate the migraine sufferer, as well as other strong scents and odors, including incense and potpourri.

Integrative (or Alternative) Treatments

In 2002, a government survey of approximately 31,000 individuals found that one-third of Americans engage in integrative or alternative medicine, which is broadly defined as any healing practice "that does not fall within the realm of conventional medicine." It is based on historical or cultural traditions, rather than on scientific evidence. Aromatherapy, chiropractic, hypnotherapy, massage, reflexology, and yoga are examples of these healing practices, and can all be beneficial to the headache patient. While there may be no (or very little) scientific evidence to support these practices, studies show that many people find them very effective for a wide range of maladies. Just as headache triggers vary from one individual to the next, alternative treatments may be effective for some patients and not for others. The key is to keep an open mind and find what works for you. Let's take a look at a few of the more popular alternative healing practices.

Yoga

Like other forms of exercise, yoga can be beneficial to the headache patient in two ways: reducing stress and improving flexibility and strength, which in turn, improves posture. Because yoga combines breathing techniques with poses that require concentration, it creates a mind-body connection that has been shown to promote relaxation and reduce stress—which is helpful in the fight against headaches. Studies show that it also releases endorphins, neurotransmitters that promote a feeling of well-being. In addition, as we discussed earlier, increased flexibility or range of motion in the back, shoulders, and neck, as well as correct alignment of the spine, are key to headache management. Yoga can be used to achieve both.

Chiropractic Care

Physicians can have widely differing opinions on the use of chiropractic techniques. While some people have found relief from back and neck pain, as well as headaches, it is important to discuss the use of chiropractic care and any manipulation of the neck with your physician. There is some risk for certain medical conditions, including stroke. Improper manipulation can also make the situation worse. The best approach is to include your chiropractor as part of your headache care team. Chiropractors may be helpful in relieving neck spasm and tension, and provide therapeutic benefits for those patients who have headaches that involve the neck (see the sidebar on Trigger Point Therapy in this chapter).

For patients who have injured their neck, back, or shoulders, and are experiencing headaches as a result of those injuries, I recommend a consultation with your doctor and physical therapy.

Thermal Biofeedback

According to the U.S. Headache Consortium, a popular behavioral therapy used in the treatment of migraine is thermal biofeedback. This is the process of training yourself to relax when you are under stress, instead of responding with the fight-or-flight reaction. It combines modern electrical technology with ancient Eastern practices and psychology. Devices are used to carefully monitor certain bodily functions like blood pressure, temperature, muscle tension, and brainwave activity—functions of which people are typically unaware. Using a finger thermometer and listening to a visualization CD-ROM that directs a person into relaxing both the mind and body, the goal of thermal biofeedback is to warm the finger temperature to 96 degrees Fahrenheit (a person experiencing a migraine often has a finger temperature in the 70s, which indicates a high stress load). By relaying the information back to the patient, biofeedback enables them to learn to control previously involuntarily-controlled body functions. Control of bodily functions can be traced back to the psychological self-discipline practices of yogis and Zen masters in Eastern cultures. Such control has been shown to be quite useful in treating headaches. The biofeedback technique is practiced on a regular basis by certified headache centers, with positive results. Details of how to obtain a finger thermometer and a CD-ROM are available at www.headachecare.com.

Prayer and Meditation

Regardless of your religious or spiritual beliefs, studies show that prayer and/or meditation can lower blood pressure, reduce stress and relieve pain. Spending just 10–20 minutes each day focusing on whatever is meaningful to you can help you relax, find balance, and regain a sense of control in a chaotic world. I have found this to be true, both personally and professionally.

Vitamins and Supplements

Although I am not a big advocate of vitamins and supplements, there is some evidence to suggest they may be helpful in managing headaches. Certainly, I have no problem with taking a daily multivitamin for overall health, since we could all use some help getting the recommended daily allowances of many nutrients. I would, however, recommend staying away from megavitamins, protein supplements and energy boosters, which may do more harm than good.

Minerals such as calcium and potassium, which may be part of a daily multivitamin, have been beneficial to some headache patients. There is also evidence that magnesium and riboflavin (vitamin B2) may reduce the frequency and severity of headaches. Coenzyme Q10, which is a nutritional supplement, has also been effective in lessening migraine attacks in some patients. However, use of these supplements can require patients to add several pills a day to an already-full pill regimen; therefore, I designed a capsule that contains all three entities, magnesium, riboflavin and Coenzyme Q10. One or two capsules a day supplies the necessary levels of all three. See the References section at the end of the book for more information on this vitamin capsule.

Vitamin B12, in the form of hydroxocobalamin, when taken intranasally (nasal spray), can also be helpful. However, before you begin taking any vitamin or supplement, consult with your physician for the proper combinations and dosages, particularly if you have other health concerns. As far as herbal supplements and all-natural remedies that promise to "cure" your headaches, my advice is to steer clear of them. There is no magic cure for headaches. If it sounds too good to be true, it probably is.

Acupressure

Used for thousands of years in China, acupressure applies the same principles as acupuncture, but without the needles, to aid relaxation and promote wellness. Acupressure practitioners use their fingers, palms, elbows, feet, or special devices to apply pressure to acupoints (or pressure points) on the body. According to traditional Chinese medical theory, these special acupoints that lie along meridians, or channels, in our body connect specific organs and pain centers. You can practice a simpler form of acupressure at home by applying gentle, steady rotating pressure to areas such as the forehead and temple with your index finger and/or thumb. Maintain that pressure for 7 to 15 seconds, and then release. Repeat as often as needed.

Stretching, deep breathing, ice packs, warm showers, massage, and other relaxation techniques can all be used to effectively ward off or reduce the severity of a headache. Again, the point is to find the methods that work best for you. It's also important to recognize the headache warning signs we discussed and take control of the situation as early as possible.

Trigger Point Therapy

In my opinion, "trigger points" may play a greater role in the perpetuation of migraines than previously thought. Trigger points are thought to be tender areas in the cells of the muscles where blood flow is reduced and metabolic waste is collected, thereby hindering the exchange of oxygen and nutrients which aid the muscle cells. Here's how it works: When our muscles contract, nerve endings release a neurotransmitter called acetylcholine, which tells the cell to release calcium and causes the muscle to contract. When the contraction is no longer needed, the acetylcholine is no longer released, and the calcium is returned to the cell, causing the muscle to relax. If this process is disturbed, the muscle may remain in a state of contraction, which in turn impedes the flow of nutrients and oxygen to the cell. Tight contraction leads to trigger points, or tender lumps, which activate neurotransmitters that send pain impulses to the neck, spinal cord, and higher centers of the brain.

Trigger points are like cult recruiters—they tend to cluster or combine, and then enlist other cells in the form of palpable nodules or knots in the tissue. These knots are tender to touch or massage and can refer pain to other parts of the body. In the case of headaches, the trigger points are often found in the trapezius muscles along the shoulders and the upper back. I also see migraine patients with trigger points along the posterior portion of the neck and areas of the jaw, which cause pain and stiffness, along with headaches. Compressing certain trigger points will actually mimic a headache, or, according to some patients, cause throbbing in the area where their headaches usually occur.

Almost all the patients I see with migraines have trigger points with referred pain patterns. In addition, the number of trigger points that a person has in his or her muscles seem to correspond to the length of a person's history with migraines and frequency of attacks. If the migraines and trigger points are not treated, then a greater number of trigger points will form and headaches will increase, producing a vicious cycle. Trigger points can also cause other symptoms, such as dizziness, vertigo, and fatigue. However, treating the various trigger points can actually prevent other trigger points from forming, and decrease the frequency and severity of migraines.

How are trigger points formed? Certainly trigger points can form after a sudden trauma or injury, but most often they develop gradually over time. Emotional factors, such as anxiety and depression, sleep problems, certain infections, and even nutritional deficiencies can lead to the formation of trigger points. Sometimes, other medical conditions contribute to the problem.

Trigger points that cause migraines need to be treated acutely by injections for a period of time, as determined by your physician. Patients receive injections at the site of the trigger point, followed by gentle, steady pressure for up to a minute. The use of acupressure, massage and gentle stretching of the muscles can also be beneficial between injections. At home, try lying on a firm bed or floor with your knees bent and placing a tennis ball under the area of the trigger point (but not the spine itself).

Hold that pressure for at least ten seconds, but not more than a minute. Then, slowly roll the ball to another area, and repeat the process. Use only one ball, not two. Mild to moderate pressure seems to work best. For trigger points that are high in your trapezius muscle on the top of your shoulders, you can gently pinch the muscle between your second or third finger and your thumb, continuing along the neck to the shoulder. Another helpful technique is moving your head slowly forward and backwards, as if you were nodding "yes," and then moving your head to the left and right, as if you were nodding "no," and finally looking straight ahead and moving your head from one shoulder to the other.

Some people find that massage helps, but if it produces severe pain, do not continue it. This will only recruit more trigger points in the future and make the problem worse. Warm showers or the application of a heating pad for 15 minutes will also help relax the muscles, and can be particularly helpful prior to injection treatment.

As with all headaches, reducing stress, seeking treatment for anxiety and depression, and regulating sleep patterns are necessary to help break the cycle of trigger point migraines. Certain substances, such as alcohol, tobacco, and marijuana aggravate trigger points and should be discontinued. Following the low-tyramine diet, outlined in this chapter, will also help. In other words, trigger point therapy involves a combination of treatments to be successful. And, when the headaches begin to resolve, treatment of trigger points should continue.

CHAPTER 5

Taking Control Part II— Medication

So, you've followed the migraine prevention diet, reduced other avoidable triggers, and made some positive lifestyle changes—and you're still plagued by persistent headaches. It may be time to consider migraine medication. Is there a magic bullet that miraculously cures headaches? No, but there are some effective medications that have provided relief to many people—and may even feel a bit like magic! Just as triggers can be unique to each headache sufferer, medication can affect people very differently. Finding the right medication, or sometimes a combination of medications, often involves trial and error. The most important point I will make regarding medication, however, is that *it must be used properly to be effective*. For instance, preventive medications must be taken daily, while acute medications must be taken in the earliest stages of a headache. And the overuse of medication will only make the situation worse (see Rebound Headaches).

And whatever you do, don't stop following the migraine diet, avoiding triggers, exercising, or engaging in other stress reduction habits. While this program may not be sufficient to control your headaches, it is a necessary part of your treatment plan. Medications are not cure-alls. They are much more effective when used in conjunction with other preventive measures.

Before we look at treatment options, I would like to discuss a common problem with medications: rebound headaches.

"I was digging myself into a hole."

Beth is 35 years old and gets headaches around her menstrual cycle that last three to four days. She has suffered from these headaches as long as she can remember, but they seemed to increase in frequency and severity when she was in her twenties. She used to take analgesics only during this three-to-four-day period, which successfully relieved her headaches. However, as her headaches became more frequent, she was eventually taking medication about half the days of the month with less relief. When simple OTC medications, such as acetaminophen and ibuprofen no longer worked, she resorted to taking combinations of medications, including aspirin with caffeine. When these failed to completely alleviate her headaches, she got a prescription for butalbital (commonly known as Fiorinal).

As Beth can testify, rebound does not happen overnight. It's typically produced over months or even years. Over time, the episodic headaches that once occurred a couple of times each month started to get worse and strike a couple of times a week, requiring more and more pain medications (and caffeine) to cope. Without realizing it, you begin digging yourself into a hole that becomes deeper and deeper.

That hole can be made even deeper by other habits. Beth was also drinking up to 24 ounces of coffee each day, as well as a large diet soda, which contains artificial sweetener. Even on the butalbital every other day, Beth was still missing work three to four days each month, and could be frequently found on the couch, holding her head and asking her children to keep the noise down. The first course of action was to remove all caffeine and artificial sweeteners from Beth's diet. To help her discontinue all previous medications, I placed her on a steroid bridge therapy and prescribed a preventive migraine medication. I also suggested a non-steroidal anti-inflammatory drug (NSAID) in place of the Fiorinal to take when a headache occurred. Her headaches steadily improved over the next six weeks, and are now manageable enough for her to go to work and enjoy her family.

Rebound Headaches

Most of the patients I see for headache consultation and treatment are already on many medications, including over-the-counter (OTC) and prescription medications, and have some component of rebound headaches. Rebound is a term we use when a headache returns with the use of an analgesic or pain medication designed to treat headaches. For the most part, analgesics or pain medication will work fairly well when used *infrequently*. However, when headaches occur more than twice a week with the use of medication, or your headache returns as soon as the medication wears off or shortly after, then you are probably experiencing rebound. Unfortunately, this creates a vicious cycle.

As your headaches continue, you resort to taking the medication more frequently, or increasing the dosage. Your headache may persist at a low level of severity even after taking the painkillers. It never completely goes away. If you don't take the medication, the headache becomes even more severe, and may become unbearable; so, of course, you take more medication. Soon you are relying on medication to get through the day. Taking more medication only complicates the situation and makes matters worse.

I am going to tell you something you don't want to hear: to stop your pain, you must stop taking the analgesic medication now. You'll notice I didn't say "stop taking it a little at a time" or "only use it when you have a severe headache." Stop taking it completely … right now! You might say, "I can't do that; I have to take medication to work!" I understand, but the reality is the only way to stop this cycle is to break it. Patients may have the worst several days, or weeks, in their lives when they withdraw from these medications, but afterward they tell me how good they feel and wonder why they didn't stop taking them earlier. **One very important note: before discontinuing any medication, you should consult with your physician, who can provide guidance on tapering off addictive medications or provide alternative medication for pain relief in the interim process.**

By far, the most common medications that lead to rebound headaches are overused analgesics which contain caffeine, such as Excedrin, Anacin, and similar OTC drugs. The caffeine in these drugs temporarily constricts the blood vessels, which have become swollen due to migraine, and therefore provide relief in the short term. However, when the drug wears off, the blood vessels react by swelling to an even greater degree—a process called *rebound vasodilation*. On the other hand, when used appropriately for *occasional* episodic headaches, these drugs work well.

The prescription migraine drugs Fiorinal and Fioricet also contain caffeine and therefore may also cause rebound (as well as addiction). However, these particular medications should not be discarded. When

Medication that May Cause Rebound Headaches

Analgesics with caffeine	Anacin, Excedrin, Esgic Plus, Fiorinal, Fioricet, B.C. Headache Powder, Vanquish, and others
Butalbital compounds	Esgic Plus, Fioricet, Fiorinal, Phrenilin, and others
Decongestants	Afrin, Dristan, Sudafed, Tylenol Sinus, and others
Ergotamines	DHE 45, Ergomar, Migranal, and Wigraine
Isometheptene compounds	Duradrin, Midrin, and others
Opioids and related narcotics	Darvocet, Percocet, OxyContin, Stadol NS, Tylenol with codeine, Ultram, and others
Triptans	Amerge, Axert, Imitrex, Maxalt, Relpax, Zomig, and others

used diligently in patients who have episodic headaches (one to three per month), these prescription medications can be extremely helpful. It's only when these drugs fail to completely alleviate the headache, or headaches last longer, or are not being relieved at all, that it's time to consider the rebound effect.

Rebound headaches can also be caused by decongestants and other related medications. Like medications with caffeine, these drugs also constrict blood vessels and provide temporary relief. Sometimes patients who mistakenly believe they are suffering from sinus head-aches will begin using decongestants, such as Sudafed, Mucinex, or Afrin nasal spray, or medications that com-bine a painkiller with a decongestant. The potential for rebound headaches occurs when the patient finds him-self having to take these medications more and more often, with lesser results, and eventually receives little or no relief. Again, the only solution is to stop taking them altogether.

If it becomes too difficult to stop taking a medication cold turkey, your doctor may prescribe a fast tapering dose of steroids, along with a different type of medica-tion, such as an NSAID (i.e., ibuprofen or naproxen) which handles the pain and inflammation of a migraine while easing you away from the medication you are trying to stop taking. Your doctor may also prescribe a preventive migraine medication which has little or no rebound effect. (We will discuss preventive medica-tions later in this chapter.) However, even triptans (i.e., Imitrex, Amerge, Zomig, Maxalt, Axert, and Relpax), which are the major drugs used to treat acute migraine headaches, can potentially cause rebound when used more than 4–6 times per month.

Additionally, narcotics or opioids, including Tylenol with codeine, Darvocet, Percocet, Stadol NS, OxyCon-tin, and oxycodone, may cause a compounded problem. Not only do patients who take these drugs risk develop-ing rebound, they must continually increase the dosage and frequency of these medications because they are habit-forming. Eventually these patients find that their doctors will not prescribe as much medication as they need to alleviate their headache pain. Again, the solution is to stop taking these medications completely, ***with the advice of your physician,*** and then work with him or her to develop an effective treatment plan. **Keep in mind, it may require in-patient or hospital treatment to successfully discontinue taking these stronger, addictive medications.** Because of this, I generally do not advocate

Signs of Rebound Headache

- *Your headaches are increasing in frequency; headaches occur more than two times per week.*
- *You have increased your use of analgesic medications without relief, and are missing work, school, or social engagements even with the use of medication.*
- *Your headaches began to change—for example, a one-sided headache becomes more diffuse across the entire head.*
- *There is less phonophobia and photophobia, and perhaps less nausea along with your headaches.*
- *The headache is developing at the same time each day, and may even occur at night.*
- *You are getting less relief from the medication you are taking, even at a stronger dose.*
- *Preventive migraine medications do not work.*

codeine, barbiturates, oxycodone, or morphine deriva-
tives for the treatment of headaches.

You Are in Control

Isn't it true that you've tried everything else? You've
tried decreasing your medication, and it didn't work.
You've tried different or stronger medications, which
may have helped slightly, but eventually your headaches
increased in frequency and severity. You may have even
gone to the ER in desperation and asked for a shot to
just "knock you out." Indeed, a good sleep can sometimes relieve a bad headache. But what happens in the
future, as you depend on these "quick fixes" of painkillers, is that your body becomes used to them. The receptor sites in your brain become like Pac-men, devouring
these medications and then craving more and more each
time the drugs are used. Sooner or later, you develop
rebound, in which not taking the medication or reducing the dose actually causes your headache to return.
To make matters worse, you may have also developed
stomach problems, which are probably side effects from
taking ibuprofen, naproxen sodium, or some combination of medications.

You may be wondering if you can ever take these
analgesics or other medications again, and the answer
is yes, you can. Once you are free of headaches for a
period of time, and/or develop headaches fewer than two

times per week, you can reintroduce these medications, and they will help alleviate your occasional headaches at that time. If the medications are taken more than two times per week, however, the rebound recurs, and you are back where you started.

The bottom line is: you must be in control of your headaches, and your life. It may sound trite, but having a positive attitude can go a long way toward overcoming any situation, including this one. I have found that migraine patients are typically very smart individuals. They tend to be compulsive at what they do. They want to do a good job. So, now it's time to do a good job for yourself. If migraines are taking over your life, and your headaches are controlling you, it's time for you to take back control. And, the first step might be stopping all pain medications—for the time being. It may be one of the hardest things you do in your life, but I can assure you it will be the most rewarding when you get your life back!

Now, you might be asking, "But what about my doctor? He keeps giving me these medications. If they are causing rebound, then why in the world would he continue to prescribe them?" When you first visit your doctor, he or she is looking for the easiest solution to your headache problem, which often involves analgesics and other pain medications to provide relief. As you continue to complain of headaches, or that your headaches are getting worse, he or she will typically prescribe different medications, hoping these will help. When these fail to work, your doctor may begin to be concerned about drug overuse, or become uncomfortable with the situation and reluctant to prescribe more medication, inadvertently making things worse. Also, some physicians may be unwilling or unable to say no to their patients' constant requests. In the end, *you* have to make the decision to stop all the medications that are causing rebound, and start working toward a better solution.

Acute Migraine Medications

When used properly, there are many medications that can effectively treat headaches. Medications for migraines are divided into two groups: acute and preventative. Acute medications treat a migraine attack after it starts. These medications are taken as soon as a patient feels a headache coming on. Preventive medications protect the nervous system from being prone to migraine and are taken daily, whether a headache is present or not. We'll begin by discussing acute medications.

About 90 percent of migraine sufferers take some form of acute medication for their attacks. The definition of acute here is "short term," meaning you take these medications for each individual migraine attack. As we discussed in the section on rebound, acute medications can make your headaches worse when used too frequently, and can actually transform an episodic migraine into a chronic daily headache. However, when used properly, these medications can offer effective relief to most patients.

Analgesics

The most common medications used to treat headaches are analgesics, commonly referred to as painkillers. Analgesics can be non-narcotic, such as OTC brands of aspirin, acetaminophen, or NSAIDs such as ibuprofen; or narcotic, such as prescription drugs containing codeine or morphine. Using painkillers *infrequently*—**no more than two days per week** for mild-to-moderate headaches—is fine, if they work. However, if your headaches are more frequent or more severe, or if these medications become causing rebound, then the focus should be on *preventing* your headaches (see Preventive Medications).

Pain medications do very little for the etiology or origin of a headache. They just dull the pain and act as a Band-Aid that keeps the headache under control, most of the time. They don't completely relieve the headache. NSAIDs, such as ibuprofen, have two effects: pain relief and anti-inflammation, at higher doses. Why is that important? Because migraines are thought to be caused by an increase or decrease of neurotransmitters in the brain, as well as inflammation. Therefore, drugs that have an anti-inflammatory property may be more effective. With NSAIDs, you need to take a higher dose to

Acute Treatment of Mild-to-Moderate Headache

Acetaminophen (without caffeine)	1,000 mg per day, or more with your doctor's advice
Aspirin (without caffeine)	1,000 mg per day, or more with your doctor's advice
Ibuprofen	Maximum of 2,400 mg per day, with your doctor's advice
Naproxen sodium	Maximum of 1,650 mg per day with your doctor's advice

(Note: All dosages should be determined by a physician who knows the patient's medical history, including other possible health issues, and individual tolerance. To avoid rebound, these drugs should be taken no more than two days per week.)

achieve this effect. So, taking 200 mg of ibuprofen, every 4–6 hours, may take the edge off your headache, but won't help the underlying problem. On the other hand, taking 600–800 mg of ibuprofen could do the trick by relieving both pain and inflammation.

The table above shows the acute treatment options for mild-to-moderate migraines. These medications should stop the headache pain once it has begun and prevent its progression—and have the least chance of rebound, when taken properly. One important point: **any medication that is given for the acute treatment of migraines should be taken early in the process of the headache to be effective.** As soon as you feel a headache coming on, before the pounding and sensitivity to light or sound begins, take the medication in a high enough dose to completely resolve the headache.

Keep in mind these medications are not without potential side effects. Aspirin, ibuprofen, and naproxen can cause stomach irritation, gastric burning and/or bleeding, or kidney problems, especially in patients who already have kidney problems or are predisposed by an underlying condition. Acetaminophen at high doses may cause liver damage. If you have chronic problems such as diabetes or high blood pressure, you should follow the advice of your physician when taking these medications.

And, don't just rely on taking medication when a headache begins. Help the medication do its job by relaxing or lying down in a quiet room, applying heat or ice, using gentle massage, or doing the neck exercises we discussed. Find what works best for you and do it as soon as a headache begins.

"I can't keep the medicine down."

Lisa is a 23-year-old who suffers from episodic migraines. About five times a month, she wakes up with a dull, pounding headache, and then becomes quite nauseous. The treatment plan developed by her doctor included taking oral migraine medication as early as possible after her headache starts. However, this plan doesn't work very well for Lisa for two reasons: 1) Since she wakes up with pain, the headache has already been in progress for some time; 2) She often vomits up her medication before it has a chance to work. Trying multiple medications at the same time also was not successful.

The goal of migraine medications is to allow the patient to function as quickly as possible—ideally, within two hours. But if a patient is unable to take a medication early on or keep a medication in his or her system, it's impossible for the medication to be absorbed properly and alleviate the headache. Oral tablets were obviously not the answer for Lisa. So, what do we do for patients like her?

We can try prescribing migraine medication in a nasal spray. Nasal sprays have the ability to be rapidly absorbed, but some is swallowed and most of the absorption occurs in the gastrointestinal tract, so there is still the potential for nausea and vomiting in some patients. Unfortunately, that was the case with Lisa. The next step might be to try injections. Injections, although painful, provide patients with rapid and reliable relief. But what if you are afraid of needles like many people, including Lisa?

Thankfully, there are now several alternative delivery options for migraine medications, including rectal delivery, needle-less injection, iontophorectic patch, and, most recently, inhaled. At present, a DHE (dihydroergotamine) is available in an inhalant, which can be taken either intranasally or through the mouth (like an asthma inhaler). In addition, a sumatriptan (Sumavel) is available in a needleless injection. This method bypasses the stomach and places the medicine directly into the system, relieving the headache quickly. This method proved highly effective for Lisa, who was able to use this injection as soon as she woke up with a headache, despite her nausea.

Triptans and Opioids

If your headaches are moderate to severe, you may need more than an analgesic. Triptans, which are drugs specifically designed for migraines, can offer effective relief for moderate to severe headaches. Again, they should not be taken more than two days per week, or they could lead to rebound. Triptans work by stimulating the neurotransmitter serotonin, and may interrupt the migraine mechanism. They have a modulating effect on the neurotransmitters, as well as an anti-inflammatory effect. Like analgesics, they should be taken at the first sign of a headache.

Triptans come in several forms (see the following table), including tablets, nasal spray, and injections. Different forms vary in their effectiveness and are better tolerated from one person to another, so you may have to try more than one to find relief. Also, for patients who are experiencing nausea along with their headache, the nasal spray or injection form may be preferable. If a headache lasts for a prolonged period, more than one dose may be required. For some patients, mixing the effects of a triptan and an NSAID provides more complete relief.

Acute Treatment of Moderate-to-Severe Headaches

Triptans

Almotriptan (Axert)	6.25 or 12.5 mg tablet
Eletriptan (Relpax)	40 to 80 mg tablet
Frovatriptan (Frova)	2.5 mg tablet
Naratriptan (Amerge)	1 or 2.5 mg tablet
Rizatriptan (Maxalt)	5 to 10 mg tablet
Sumatriptan (Imitrex)	25, 50 or 100 mg tablet
Sumatriptan (Imitrex)	5 or 25 mg nasal spray
Sumatriptan	4 or 6 mg self-injection
Zolmitriptan (Zomig)	2.5 or 5 mg tablet

Non-triptans

DHE (dihydroergotamine mesylate)	1 mg intravenous, subcutaneous or nasal spray

Opioids

Codeine	30 to 60 mg orally
Oxycodone	5 to 10 mg orally

(Note: Dosages are determined by a physician and are based on the height/weight, medical history and individual tolerance of the patient. When used more than two days per week, triptans and opioids can cause rebound, and opioids can become habit-forming.)

Like most medications, triptans do carry the risk of certain side effects. While the tablet form is usually well tolerated, the injectable form can cause dizziness, flushing, numbness, tingling, and tightness of the throat or chest. Though these side effects are fairly common, the injectable form may still be preferred because it works faster. In rare cases, triptans can cause serious complications, especially in patients who have coronary artery disease. These medications should never be taken without the advice and supervision of a physician.

For patients who are at risk for complications from triptans, or don't respond well to them, an opioid such as codeine or oxycodone may be a better choice. As I have said, these drugs are narcotics and can be habit-forming, as well as lead to rebound. They should not be used more than two days per week, and only under the supervision of a physician.

For some people, triptans can actually make the nausea associated with a migraine worse. If that's the case, or you are having difficulty keeping the medication down, there are a number of anti-nausea drugs available that can be taken in conjunction with triptans (see the following table). These drugs can be administered orally, or if nausea and vomiting are severe, by injection or rectally. Because anti-nausea drugs block the action of the neurotransmitter dopamine, they can not only relieve nausea and vomiting, but also help relieve the headache, and they don't cause rebound. Therefore,

Treatment of Nausea and Vomiting

Metoclopramine (Reglan)	10 to 20 mg up to 4 times daily	Injection or orally
Prochlorperazine (Compazine)	5 to 10 mg up to 3 or 4 times daily	Orally or injection
	25 mg up to twice daily	Rectally
Promethazine (Phenergan)	12.5 to 25 mg up to every 4 hours	Orally, by injection, or rectally
Trimethobenz-amide (Tigan)	250 mg up to 3 or 4 times daily	Orally
	200 mg up to 3 to 4 times daily	Rectally

(Note: Dosages are determined by a physician and are based on the height/weight, medical history, and individual tolerance of the patient.)

they may help a patient who is trying to discontinue analgesics due to rebound.

When choosing which acute medication to use, a physician should consider the frequency and severity of your migraine attacks, as well as any accompanying symptoms, such as nausea. An effective treatment plan may involve a step approach, using more than one medication. For instance, it may start with an analgesic (painkiller), combined with an anti-nausea drug. If that doesn't work, a triptan may be prescribed, along with a "rescue drug," such as an opioid for a severe migraine attack. As mentioned before, a combination of an NSAID and a triptan can also be very effective for some patients. The physician must work along with the patient to find the formula that works best for each individual case. This process may take weeks or even months until an effective combination is found. It's important for patients to not get frustrated and lapse from care during that period. And, once this formula is discovered it should be monitored very carefully to avoid rebound and other complications.

Another method of treatment is stratified care. With this approach, patients are assessed to determine the severity or level of disability associated with their migraines, and medication is then prescribed based on that assessment. In other words, each patient may begin with a different "step." So, for instance, a patient with a mild headache and no disability can initially be managed with OTC drugs, while a patient with moderate headaches may need an analgesic together with an antinausea medication. For those headache sufferers who have a significant disability, we may start with an acute medication approved to treat moderate to severe headaches, such as a triptan or DHE. Again, it may take several office visits and several medication changes to find relief.

How do you know when to change your acute medication? Ask yourself these questions:

- Does my medication work consistently in the majority of my migraine attacks?
- Does the headache pain disappear within two hours?
- Am I able to function normally within two hours after taking the medication?
- Am I comfortable enough with this medication to be able to plan my daily activities without fear of a headache?

One or more "no" answers may indicate a need to change your treatment plan—and it may be time to consider preventive medication.

Let's Review:

- Used too frequently (more than two days a week), pain medications can cause rebound headaches.
- The only way to stop rebound headaches is to completely stop taking the medication that is causing the rebound.
- When used properly, analgesics and NSAIDs can alleviate infrequent mild-to-moderate headaches.
- Triptans can be very effective at treating moderate to severe headaches, when taken as prescribed.
- Acute migraine medications should be taken at the first sign of a headache, and are more effective when the patient assists the medication by relaxing or lying down.

Preventive Migraine Medications

If your headaches are too frequent, too severe, or too long-lasting to be relieved by acute medications, you may be a candidate for preventive migraine medications. Preventive or prophylactic medications are usually taken daily to protect the patient from having a migraine. Remember, migraine-prone individuals have a sensitive nervous system and a low threshold for potential triggers. Preventive medication essentially raises your threshold level. In other words, they stop your glass from spilling over so easily.

These medications are classified into three categories:

- Beta-blockers (also used for high blood pressure)
- Antidepressants
- Anticonvulsants

As you can see, these medications were not originally designed to treat migraines, but over time we have found them to be effective in the prevention of migraine in some people. Don't be confused: just because your doctor prescribes an antidepressant for your migraines, it doesn't mean that he or she thinks you are suffering from depression. Migraines are associated with a sensitive nervous system and the fluctuations of neurotransmitters, which these drugs also affect. By blocking or enhancing certain neurotransmitters, these drugs make the migraine mechanism harder to trigger, or less fully activated when it is triggered. However, the dosage of these medications, when used to treat migraine, is typically lower than the dose given for the condition the medication was intended to treat.

If you start taking preventive medication, you might wonder if you will have to take it forever. Not necessarily. Once the frequency of your headaches decreases and stabilizes over a period of time (usually three to six months), the medication can be tapered off. If the headaches get worse, then treatment is resumed. If headaches stay under control, the medication can be discontinued. Your physician can work with you to find the right dosage and treatment plan over time.

Although preventive medications raise your migraine threshold, that doesn't mean you can stop avoiding migraine triggers! On the contrary, these medications work best when patients eliminate or reduce dietary triggers, and engage in the other migraine prevention behaviors we've talked about earlier. The more you avoid migraine triggers, the less preventive medication you will need to take. Think of it as a comprehensive treatment plan.

As with other drugs, you may have to try more than one preventive medication to find one that works best for you. Your physician will typically start you at the lowest possible dosage in order to avoid potential side effects, and then slowly increase it over time until your

Preventive Migraine Medication

Medication	Dosages	Other conditions treated	Possible Side Effects
Beta-Blockers—		High blood pressure and certain heart conditions	Fatigue, insomnia, depression; may be a problem with asthma or diabetes
Nadolol (Corgard)	40–80 mg daily		
Propanolol (Inderal)	240 mg daily		
Timolol (Blocadren)	5–30 mg daily		
Calcium Channel Blockers—		High blood pressure	Constipation
Verapamil (Calan)	80–120 mg three times a day		
Diltiazam (Cardizem)	30–90 mg three times a day		
Corticosteroids—		Useful for brief treatment of "crises"	Many side effects, especially if used long-term
Prednisone	20–80 mg daily		

Drug	Dosage	Uses	Side effects
Antihistamines—			
Cyproheptadine (Periactin)	4–16 mg daily	Antihistamine for allergies	Sedation, increased appetite
Anticonvulsives—			
Divalproex (Depakote)	150–500 mg twice daily	Seizures, manic-depressive illness	Nausea, tremor, hair loss, sedation, increased appetite
Topirimate (Topamax)	5–100 mg twice daily	Seizures (antiepilepsy)	Sedation, dizziness, confusion
Tricyclic antidepressants—			
Amitriptyline (Elavil)	10–300 mg at bedtime	Insomnia, depression, anxiety	Dry mouth, sedation, constipation, increased appetite
Nortriptyline (Pamelor)	10–150 mg at bedtime		

(Note: Dosages should be determined by a physician based on the height/weight, medical history and individual tolerance of the patient.)

headaches are under control. It can take some time to find the right dosage—one that controls headaches with minimal side effects—so patience is often required for successful treatment. Don't be automatically discouraged by initial side effects, such as dry mouth or fatigue, because these will often diminish over time.

There are many options to choose from when it comes to preventive migraine medications. When prescribing a particular medication, your doctor should consider any other health issues you may have, such as high blood pressure, heart conditions, insomnia, or anxiety. It is not uncommon for migraines to go hand-in hand with depression or anxiety, which we will discuss in more detail in Chapter 6. If this is the case, then some preventive medications will work effectively on both conditions. If there are no other health issues, it's often a matter of choosing a preventive medication that causes the least side effects and works best for that particular patient.

What if a migraine "breaks through" while you are on preventive medication? You can take a triptan or an occasional painkiller when this happens. Just be careful not to get back on the slippery slope of rebound!

Why Not Just Start With Preventive Medication?

Although preventive migraine medications are generally safe for long-term use, most people would prefer not to take any medication on a daily basis if it can be avoided. All medications have potential risks and side effects. And many migraine patients do not need to use preventive medications. If we start with preventive medications we will never know if lifestyle changes or the occasional use of acute medication will be effective. We may also never discover the origin or source of the headache. Therefore, we typically begin treatment with the most important and basic step—lifestyle changes such as diet, exercise, and relaxation techniques. These are the foundation of all other treatments.

When lifestyle changes fail to control your headaches, the next step is the occasional use of acute medications,

---

Let's Review:

- Preventive migraine medications raise your migraine threshold and must be taken daily.

- Avoiding migraine triggers and maintaining positive lifestyle changes will make these medications work more effectively and require a smaller dosage.

- It may take several months and some adjustments to dosage to achieve success with preventive medications.

- Choosing a preventive medication will depend on any coexisting health conditions, as well as your tolerance to possible side effects.

and finally we move to preventive medications, when necessary.

Take Your Medicine

Mary Poppins once said, "A spoonful of sugar helps the medicine go down," but if you're suffering from nausea and vomiting—common complaints with migraine patients—it's sometimes impossible to take your medicine and keep it down. Thankfully, there are alternate delivery systems for migraine medication, including some that are still in development. First, let's take a look at the advantages and disadvantages of currently available delivery systems:

1. *Oral tablets—These are preferred by many patients, but absorption may be impaired if you have nausea or vomiting. You may also develop gastric stasis, which is the inability of the duodenum (small intestine) to move fluids and medication through your digestive system.*
2. *Oral disintegrating tablets or wafers—Because these dissolve in your mouth, you don't need to drink water or other fluids when you take them. However, nausea and vomiting can still impair absorption.*
3. *Nasal sprays—These have the potential for rapid absorption, but even though the medication is being inhaled through the nose, most of the medication is swallowed, so absorption still occurs in your digestive system.*

---

4. Subcutaneous injections—*These are reliable and deliver medication rapidly into your system—5–10 minutes versus 30–60 minutes for oral tablets. Some people have an aversion to needles, however.*

5. Rectal—*Sumatriptan (a triptan) is available in 20 mg suppositories, which deliver the medication rectally. There are no pharmacokinetic (relating to the process by which a drug is absorbed and metabolized) differences between rectal and oral delivery.*

6. Transdermal—*Medication is delivered through a patch adhered to the skin (iontophoretic patch). This allows the medication to be absorbed directly through the skin and into the bloodstream, bypassing the digestive system.*

New and developmental delivery systems for acute treatment include:

1. Inhaled by mouth—*DHE Medication is inhaled orally in this system, and the system is also used as a delivery system for asthma or COPD inhalers, referred to as pulmonary systemic absorption. The availability of the medication inhaled through the mouth is about twice as high as the intranasal route. It bypasses the stomach completely, and begins working in 30 minutes or less.*

2. Intranasally (within the nose)—*Intranasal sumatriptan uses a breath-actuated device, which results in rapid, systemic absorption.*

3. *Needleless injections—Subcutaneous injections of sumatriptan (with needles), given by either the patient or a physician is the fastest and strongest delivery system. However, an alternative is a needle-free injection using a high-pressure nitrogen gas source, which delivers a narrow jet of sumatriptan solution through the skin. This is similar to an auto-injector or spring-loaded syringe (e.g., Epipen). It is easy to use and is intended for self-administration by patients. The site of the injection depends on the drug loaded, but it's typically administered into the thigh, buttocks, or abdomen. Relief with this method can be obtained as quickly as five to ten minutes.*

4. *Transcranial magnetic stimulation (TMS)—This delivery system is particularly useful for the relief of migraine with aura. It's a non-invasive method in which a brief magnetic pulse is delivered to the scalp and underlying cortex, altering the pattern of the nerve cells. It's thought that this pulse modulates the circuits of the brain involved in pain processing. In other words, it short-circuits the pain signal.*

If you are having trouble taking your medication due to nausea and vomiting, or need a faster delivery system, discuss these alternative delivery systems with your doctor.

CHAPTER 6

Beyond Headache

As you might expect, people with sensitive nervous systems are not only predisposed to migraines, but also prone to other health problems that share similar etiologies—that is, diseases that stem from the same cause or origin. These conditions are called *comorbid disorders*. The word "comorbid" is used to describe secondary or tertiary illnesses or disorders that exist in a person in addition to a primary illness. Depression, anxiety, hypertension, and even cardiac problems are examples of disorders that are closely associated with migraine and often occur simultaneously. When treating migraine, it's important to diagnose and treat any other medical issues that may be interacting with your headaches. As I've said before, it's essential to treat the whole person.

This chapter delves into some of the more common comorbid disorders. While I believe an informed patient is a good patient, my first word of advice is "don't be alarmed!" Just because you suffer from chronic headaches does not necessarily mean you have other medical problems or that you will eventually develop these conditions. However, if you do recognize yourself in these pages, you can use that information to your advantage. Arming yourself with knowledge can not only help you and your physician knock out headaches, it may help you prevent or treat any related disorders.

Depression

Which came first, the chicken or the egg? This age-old quandary can also be applied to the relationship between migraine and depression. Depression occurs in 25–35% of the migraine population and affects the same neurotransmitters as migraine. Neurotransmitters are substances in the body which transmit nerve impulses across the synapses (gaps) between nerve cells. In the headache sufferer, these substances are serotonin and norepinephrine. In patients with depression, the level of these substances is lower than normal, which causes the depressed patient to move more slowly, think more sluggishly, and have difficulty concentrating. Migraine itself, without depression, also lowers the levels of serotonin and norepinephrine, with the same consequences. So, you can see how the two may go hand-in-hand.

No one can say for certain what the actual cause and effect between migraine and depression really is. It's easy to understand how the chronic pain of migraine headaches can eventually lead to depression. But this process also works in reverse. Research has shown that patients who are depressed are, in fact, more likely to suffer from migraine. No matter which one comes first, recognizing the symptoms of depression and treating it is key. The following checklist can help you determine if you are suffering from depression, and may provide valuable information for your doctor:

____ Do you have little interest or pleasure in doing things you used to enjoy?

____ Do you feel down, depressed, or hopeless?

____ Do you have trouble falling asleep or staying asleep, or do you sleep too much?

____ Do you have the feeling of being tired all the time or of having little energy?

____ Has your appetite increased or decreased?

____ Do you feel bad about yourself, feel you are a failure, or that you've let your family down?

____ Do you have trouble concentrating on things such as reading the newspaper, watching TV, or performing tasks at work?

_____ Have people noticed that you are moving or speaking slowly, or conversely, that you have been fidgety or restless, and moving around more than usual?

_____ Do you ever have thoughts about hurting yourself or that you would be better off dead?

_____ Do you find yourself crying or on the verge of tears for no reason?

If you answered "yes" to three or more of these questions, particularly the first two, it's time to talk to your doctor about treatment for depression. Although closely intertwined, the symptoms of migraine and depression must be treated individually. As we saw in chapter five, some tricyclic antidepressants are used to treat migraine, and that's a good place to start. However, an antidepressant that is effective for your depression may be ineffective for migraine. Likewise, the treatment for migraine will often have little or no effect on your depression.

Many of the lifestyle changes we discussed will not only help alleviate migraines, but also help patients cope with depression and anxiety, including eating right, exercising, and adopting stress-reduction techniques. Normalizing your sleep pattern as quickly as possible is particularly important for both conditions. If you are sleeping well, then you are less tired during the day and better able to cope with life's demands, and your anxiety level will be reduced. Non-pharmacological sleep aids, such as making a habit of going to bed and getting up at the same times each day and finding a relaxing bedtime routine, should be tried first. Antidepressants will usually help a patient sleep better, but sometimes a separate medication is necessary.

A more serious and debilitating form of depression called *bipolar depression* can also be linked with migraine. This condition, which is also known as manic-depressive disorder, is characterized by alternating episodes of depression and mania, which is an abnormally elated mental state that may include feelings of euphoria, racing thoughts, lack of inhibitions, and extremely intense interests or desires. Studies suggest there is a strong genetic influence in bipolar depression, which means it tends to run in families, like migraine. This disorder typically begins in adolescence or early adulthood and continues throughout life, but there are effective treatments available.

"Headaches take the focus off my depression and anxiety."

Sally is an extreme case—one of only three or four in my career. In her 40s, she is well-educated and successful. She has several degrees from various universities and is fluent in five languages. She has traveled around the world and lived in several countries. Like many driven people, she has always been prone to headaches. Interestingly, she was able to go to many different pharmacies on her travels and obtain just about any OTC or prescription drug we have in the United States fairly easily. She kept her headaches under control by taking some type of medication on a daily basis, and was able to not only do her work, but excel at it—until the sky exploded.

Sally was part of a group of people running away from the World Trade Center on 9/11. As the building blew up and chaos ensued, she was changed irrevocably. First she developed a manic depressive–type episode, along with acute anxiety, and then became very depressed. She continues, even now, to cycle between anxiety and depression. Along with that, her headaches became more frequent and severe. Despite her education and past success, Sally is now living with her parents with no job or desire to find one. She is truly disabled at this point.

She has been non-responsive to all non-pharmacological and pharmacological treatments tried. In addition, she has been to two very well-respected headache centers and treated by some of the best headache specialists in the country, without relief. Working together with a prominent psychiatrist, we are trying to get her anxiety and depression, which has been diagnosed as post-traumatic stress syndrome, under control. It seems to both her psychiatrist and me that the headaches somehow decrease the stress and depression. It is a bit like releasing a demon trapped inside her.

Let me emphasize that Sally is a wonderful person, and someone I admire. The fact that she is extremely intelligent does make her more difficult to treat, which I have found to be true in many cases. Though we have developed a good doctor-patient partnership, it's sometimes like pulling teeth trying to get her to comply with simple orders, such as going to bed and getting up at the same time each day, or eating regular meals. Any suggestion seems to be viewed as a command which she resents. However, there has been some improvement, and I remain optimistic that we can eventually get her back on her feet and living her life to the fullest again.

Anxiety

By the time many of my patients come to see me, they are not only suffering from headaches, but are completely stressed out and want some type of medication to ease their anxiety. It's no surprise that chronic headaches can cause anxiety. If you're plagued with headaches, then chances are you are missing work, having trouble keeping up with obligations at home, sleeping poorly, and worrying about disappointing family and friends. Who wouldn't be stressed out? Under these conditions, it's not uncommon for patients to be irritable, suffer bouts of crying, or lose interest in hobbies and other activities. Remember, patients with headaches, especially migraine, have inherited a very sensitive nervous system. So, as the world moves faster and faster, and the sensory stimuli around us becomes harder to control, people with a sensitive nervous system find it more difficult to cope. You work harder and harder to keep up with deadlines and stay organized, but it seems there is not enough time in a day. Your nervous system begins to overload, which leads not only to headaches, but also anxiety. But is it anxiety or depression?

The two are often linked. Patients with depression may also have anxiety, and vice versa. Many times, I find there is a case of underlying depression in patients who come in with symptoms of anxiety, as it's often part of the depressive process. In either case, I am very cautious about prescribing anti-anxiety drugs or tranquilizers, because they can be habit-forming and cause rebound headaches, which only makes things worse. Antidepressants are typically a more effective treatment option. However, since antidepressants can take two to three weeks to begin working, in some cases anti-anxiety medications can be taken during that interim period and then slowly removed. If a patient is already taking an anti-anxiety drug, they can continue to take it while the antidepressant takes effect.

Just like migraine medications, antidepressants come in many formulas. It may take a bit of trial and error to find one that works effectively for you. My advice is the same: have patience and don't give up. Once you find the right medication, antidepressants can be very effective.

There is a helpful tool we use to determine an individual's level of stress and/or anxiety, called the Hamilton Anxiety Scale. You'll find this questionnaire at the back of the book (Appendix II). If you are feeling anxious, depressed, or stressed out due to your headaches, take a few minutes to complete this questionnaire. Again, it can provide valuable information to you and your physician as you develop a treatment plan.

Cardiac Concerns

Does your heart sometimes race or skip a beat? Anxiety often leads to excitability of the cardiac system. Skipped heartbeats, a racing heart, and pounding in the chest are common complaints of patients suffering from anxiety, as well as migraine. Even if a patient is not experiencing a true anxiety disorder, the pain of a migraine can make you anxious and affect the cardiac system. Migraine patients frequently complain of skipped heartbeats, called *premature ventricular contractures* or *premature atrial contractions*, as well as pounding in the chest. Headache sufferers will sometimes say they can hear their heart pounding loudly in their ears or head, coinciding with the throbbing of their headache. They may also experience some discomfort in the chest. While all this activity is no doubt scary and uncomfortable, it is typically benign. Getting the headache under control will usually alleviate the cardiac activity, as well.

Fibromyalgia

Often called *chronic pain syndrome*, fibromyalgia is really a hypersensitivity of nerve bundles and muscles.

It occurs mainly in the shoulders, neck, sides of the upper and lower back, wrists, ankles and feet. People with fibromyalgia say they "hurt all over." What's interesting is that the pain is out of proportion to the stimulus. In other words, a patient with fibromyalgia pain may feel like a 1,000-pound press is coming down in the area where he or she is being touched. Pulses of pain that arise from the point of contact are perceived in the brain as being much more painful than they actually are. This is caused by the hyperactivity and stimulation of the nervous system—which is where the connection with migraines comes into play.

Just as the pain of migraine is not "made up," the pain of fibromyalgia is not fabricated or exaggerated. It's very real to the person experiencing it. In both fibromyalgia and migraine, the brain perceives the pain signals in a hypersensitive state. And, as with migraine, lifestyle changes, physical therapy, and stress management can help alleviate the symptoms. In addition, there are medications available to treat fibromyalgia, including antidepressants, anticonvulsants, narcolepsy drugs, pain relievers (targeting nerve pain), and sleep aids. When used to treat fibromyalgia, these medications alter brain chemistry to help reduce pain, improve sleep, and ease anxiety or depression.

Hypertension

Hypertension, or high blood pressure, occurs when the blood pressure in the arteries is elevated. This requires the heart to work harder than normal to circulate blood through the vessels. High blood pressure can be primary, meaning there is no underlying medical cause, or secondary, which means it's caused by other conditions that affect the arteries, heart, or kidneys. Because hypertension is a major risk factor for stroke and heart attacks, it's very important to keep it under control. Dietary and lifestyle changes can improve hypertension, but drug treatment is often necessary.

Hypertension affects 1 in 4 adults in the U.S., and is seen in migraine patients fairly often. High blood pressure, in itself, can cause headaches. The good news is there are medications that can help hypertension and migraines at the same time (see Chapter 5).

Stomach/Gastrointestinal Issues

When we talk about migraine, we frequently end up talking about the stomach. Aside from the nausea associated with the headache itself, there seems to be a link between digestive issues and migraine, although it's still unclear how that link works. One problem believed to be common in migraine patients is a condition called *gastric stasis*. Gastric stasis basically means that food stays in your stomach longer than it should. This is problematic when taking oral medications for migraine, because medications are not absorbed well when they are contained in your stomach. This inability to absorb medication properly is one reason to explore the alternative medication delivery systems outlined in Chapter 5.

Another common complaint in migraine patients is *acid reflux*, which occurs when stomach acid backs up into the esophagus, causing a burning sensation. It can produce a wide range of symptoms, from heartburn (the most common), to regurgitation and difficulty swallowing. Some people may also become hoarse. Certain foods and beverages, such as hot spicy meals, onions, chocolate, coffee, tea, alcohol, and acidic fruits and juices tend to aggravate the condition and should be avoided. It's also recommended that patients with acid reflux eat smaller, more frequent meals because large meals cause the stomach to produce excess acid. Raising the upper body with pillows while sleeping can also help alleviate symptoms, as well as avoiding meals right before bedtime. It's interesting to note that some of the foods that aggravate acid reflux also trigger migraines, such as coffee, alcohol, and chocolate—yet another reason to follow the migraine prevention diet.

The link between food, digestive problems, and headaches may be stronger than we think. Some studies suggest that many digestive problems, including irritable bowel syndrome (IBS), are caused by hidden food allergies—and that food allergies can also cause migraines. If this is the case, then once the offending food(s) is discovered and removed from the diet, both the digestive distress and the headaches improve. In fact, patients with digestive problems often have other health issues, including migraines. Many of my migraine patients do suffer from excess gas, abdominal pain, bouts of constipation and diarrhea, and IBS. Again, is it the chicken or the egg first? While we don't fully understand the connection between migraine and certain digestive problems, we can treat them separately and provide relief for both. Be sure to discuss any gastrointestinal issues you are experiencing with your physician.

Also keep in mind that gastrointestinal problems can be part of the premonitory or prodrome phase of your migraine (see Chapter 2). Some migraine patients experience an upset stomach, diarrhea, a marked increase or decrease in appetite, and even cravings for certain foods prior to a migraine attack. Keeping an accurate headache diary can help you identify these often subtle changes occurring within your body that alert you to the beginning of a headache. Once alerted, you can take preventive measures.

While certain links between gastrointestinal problems and migraines are still a mystery, one thing we do know is that some medications used to alleviate headaches can cause stomach distress. Aspirin, ibuprofen, and naproxen can irritate the stomach, and with long-term use potentially result in gastric burning and/ or bleeding. In addition, some migraine-specific medications have side effects such as nausea or constipation. If you suspect your medication is causing gastrointestinal issues, talk to your doctor about changing prescriptions or adding an acid reducer, stool softener, or anti-nausea medication, as the case may be.

Dysmenorrhea

Many women who suffer from migraines also have extremely painful menstrual periods, which is a condition called *dysmenorrhea*. Their headaches also tend to become more prevalent and/or severe during menstruation. Though painful and sometimes even disabling, menstrual cramps and uterine contractions are typically benign. They can, however, be associated with a process called *endometriosis*, a medical condition in which cells from the lining of the uterus appear and flourish outside the uterine cavity, most commonly on the ovaries. These painful cysts are influenced by hormonal changes, and symptoms often worsen with the menstrual cycle. Studies have shown that using an anti-inflammatory medication, such as ibuprofen, two to three days before menstruation and then throughout the period, can help alleviate *dysmenorrhea*. Additional treatment options should be discussed with your doctor.

Fatigue

Fatigue is a natural companion to many of these comorbid problems. Migraines, anxiety, depression, fibromyalgia, and even irritable bowel syndrome can cause patients to feel worn out. In some cases, this fatigue can be so severe it causes a person to become bedridden. Patients say they don't feel like moving, or they don't have the energy to get up. This actually makes the situation worse, for muscles that aren't used become decompensated or deteriorated and weak, which makes them achier and more difficult to move. It's very important to keep the muscles active and toned, no matter how challenging it may be to muster your energy. Staying active will not only decrease muscle pain, it will help alleviate your headaches, lower blood pressure, and reduce anxiety, among other benefits.

Attention Deficit Disorder

Interestingly enough, some studies have shown that attention deficit disorder (ADD) may be an important comorbidity to migraine. It is most commonly diagnosed in children, but ADD often goes unrecognized and untreated in the adult population. Adults with this condition may be at risk for addiction to alcohol, drugs, gambling, or other compulsive behaviors. They may also have difficulty with their jobs and handling family dynamics. Patients who suffer from migraines along with ADD are at greater risk for becoming addicted to painkillers, and often require the help of both a physician who treats the headaches and a doctor who handles the psychological problem.

Post-Traumatic Headache

Sometimes patients will develop headaches following a head or neck injury. Any blow to or jarring of the head, even if it doesn't result in injury to the skull or brain, can result in residual headaches, as well as dizziness, vertigo, blurred vision, and tinnitus (ringing in the ears), as well as difficulty with memory, concentration, and attention. In some cases, the injury lowers the migraine threshold, so the patient gets headaches more easily and is more sensitive to stimuli that may trigger headaches. However, post-traumatic headaches typically resolve over time (from a couple of weeks to a couple of months), and as long as there is no injury to the brain, we treat them the same way we treat migraine. *(Note: all head and neck injuries should be seen by a physician to rule out concussion, or damage to the brain or vertebrae.)*

If you've ever been hit from behind when driving your car and experienced whiplash (a sudden, violent movement of the neck backward and forward), you know how painful it can be. Whiplash causes stretching and tearing of muscles and ligament fibers in the neck, and can sometimes lead to headaches. Again, if these headaches become chronic, we typically treat them the same way we treat migraine, with migraine-specific medications. While very uncomfortable, this type of soft-tissue injury usually gets better within a few weeks. Patients with persistent neck pain or headaches can benefit from trigger point injections and/or physical therapy.

Unfortunately, post-traumatic headaches can sometimes lead people down two dead-end roads: unnecessary surgery and prolonged litigation. I have seen many folks who, out of frustration and misdiagnosis, resort to surgery to repair a disc in the neck or have nerve ablation surgery, in which the injured nerve is blocked, only to find that their headaches are still present. The surgeries are often unsuccessful in alleviating headaches, and I would urge anyone considering surgery of this type to get a second opinion. A scan may indicate a bulging disc or pressure on a nerve, but this is often "incidental," meaning it's not the source of the headache problem.

The second dead end is found in our legal system. Post-traumatic headaches are often embellished by lawyers, and many of these cases end up in months or even years of litigation. As much as I hate to say it, when insurance companies and lawsuits are involved, a good number of these headache cases become chronic and impossible to treat. A person may be incentivized to continue having headaches until the situation is resolved. It's interesting to note that in other countries where there is litigation but no compensation after accidents, there is also a lower incidence of post-traumatic headaches.

Musculoskeletal Problems

Migraines can be a pain in the neck, literally. Almost all of my migraine patients complain about neck pain as a component of their headaches, either before, during, or after a migraine attack. This is no surprise. The neck is the cervical portion of the spine, made up of seven segments, commonly referred to as C-1 to C-7, with cartilaginous discs between each vertebra. The neck not only supports the weight of our heads, it also protects the nerves that carry sensory and motor information from the brain down to the rest of our bodies, including the trigeminal nerve. As you may recall, the trigeminal nerve plays a key role in the migraine mechanism.

Now we are back to our chicken-and-egg quandary: is the migraine causing the neck pain, or is a problem in the neck causing the migraine? It could be either. Migraine pain can affect the neck, as we've seen. On the other hand, problems in the neck can activate sensory nerves that carry signals, which act as triggers, to the migraine center in the brain, which is actually the trigeminal nucleus chordalis. So, for instance, if a patient has arthritis of the neck, which is pinching one of the nerves high in the vertebral column around C-2 and C-3, he or she will often have pain in the forehead, below the eyes or around the jaw, as well as neck pain and head-aches. Problems in the neck can also refer pain down the arms, as well as cause numbness and tingling in the arms and hands. Some pain may also occur in the shoulder or upper back area. I commonly find trigger points in these areas, which can be injected to relieve headache pain, along with pain in the affected area. The pain relief does not last, though, unless the patient does physical therapy or exercises at home to maintain flexibility.

Osteoarthritis is not always accepted as a cause of headaches, however. Almost everyone over the age of 40 has some type of osteoarthritis, but not all of these peo-ple experience headaches. As we get older, and develop more arthritis, we are prone to more problems with the neck, so it's very important to exercise and stay flex-ible. It can be tricky to diagnose, but it's important to determine the source of the headache pain in order to treat it effectively. As I mentioned before, the symptoms of migraine are often mistakenly attributed to cervical problems, which can result in unnecessary and often unreliable surgeries. Cervical spine surgery of any kind should always be a last resort.

A related issue is the *cervicogenic headache*. This is simply a fancy medical term for muscle pain in the neck that causes a headache. Many people experience this when they have a minor car accident, as we discussed earlier, but it can also occur when you've strained your neck by lifting something heavy or by sleeping in an awkward position. There are over 20 muscles in your neck that attach to the scalp and can refer pain up to the head. When these muscles are strained and continually spasm, they pull on the scalp and create pain in the head. This pain is often described as a pulling, throbbing sensation. In patients that are already prone to migraine, these spasms can provoke the problem. Treatment for *cervicogenic headaches* include: physical therapy, trigger point injections, exercise, using pillows made to support the neck and head correctly, and medication (antispasmodics or muscle relaxants).

Finally, I am often asked about a condition called *Arnold-Chiari malformation* or abnormal bones in the head and/or neck. This is a problem where the back of the brain extends downward into the spinal cord. Depending on the patient's posture, it can cause headaches, fatigue, muscle weakness in the head and face, difficulty swallowing, dizziness, nausea, impaired coordination, and, in severe cases, paralysis. Patients with this syndrome often come to see me after they have had surgery to repair the malformation, and still suffer from chronic headaches. I caution patients that surgery of this type may not be a cure-all when it comes to headaches; it should be considered only when surgery is deemed absolutely necessary due to impending neurological paralysis.

Headache Evolution

As a doctor treating headaches, I am most worried about the evolution of acute or occasional migraines becoming chronic, as headaches occur closer and closer together, until they may even be a daily event. When migraines become chronic and disabling, the condition is associated with greater comorbidity. In other words, what starts out as a headache problem becomes associated with IBS, fibromyalgia, or depression. At that point, it becomes more difficult to manage and treat, and as stated earlier, the patient no longer returns to his or her normal functioning. The patient then feels "out of control," and is more burdensome to him- or herself, and also to the healthcare system, requiring more emergency calls, doctor's visits, and disability from work. To prevent this from happening, headaches should be treated early and effectively. The idea is to reverse the process through the steps outlined in this book: understanding your headaches, making lifestyle changes, and working with your physician to find the right medication, if necessary (see the Treatment Plan Checklist in Chapter 7).

The bottom line is that you are not just a person with headaches—you are a unique biological identity consisting of approximately 100 trillion cells! Your body is made up of many complex and amazing systems, including the musculoskeletal, digestive, immune, respiratory, endocrine, and nervous systems, to name a few. These systems interact and work together, so when one system is out of balance, there's a good chance that other areas in the body are feeling the effects. Treating one aspect of a patient, without looking at the entire picture, rarely results in success, especially since migraine is a condition that impacts many aspects of your health and well-being. That's why it's so important to develop an open, honest relationship with your primary care physician—and we will discuss how to do that in the next chapter.

"Tests can be misleading."

While I believe in conducting a thorough examination and treating all aspects of my patients' health, I would like to offer a warning about over-testing—too many tests with over-interpretation of the tests performed. Conducting too many tests may reveal an abnormality that is not the source of the headache problem at all, and is usually benign.

Alice is a perfect example of the dangers inherent with excessive medical tests, and the possible misinterpretation which can produce misleading results. She came to see me with an MRI in her hand and tears in her eyes. In a frightened voice, she stated that she was diagnosed as having multiple sclerosis (MS). Naturally, she was distraught at the thought of ending up in a wheelchair, and asked me for a second opinion.

Over the past few months, she had developed numbness and tingling in her left cheek, which spread to her head, neck, and down her right arm and leg. This numbness and tingling lasted a few minutes, and then completely went away. She also had a history of headaches, and took analgesics for years to control them. The concern came when her MRI showed glistening white bodies in the brain, which could be an indication of multiple sclerosis. But these particular "spots" were not in the place we usually find them in MS. We do see these glistening white bodies in certain parts of the brain in patients who have chronic migraine headaches. A further physical exam showed that Alice was completely within normal limits and not exhibiting any pattern of symptoms seen in MS. Her symptoms were actually part of a migraine aura that lasted no more than 30 minutes before the headache. She began taking a migraine-specific medication and soon afterwards, her headaches, along with the other neurological problems she was experiencing, resolved. I'm happy to say she's been well since.

CHAPTER 7

The Patient–Doctor Partnership

It sounds easy enough: you go to the doctor because you want to get better, and your doctor prescribes some type of treatment to help you do just that. But the process is far from simple. For treatment of any kind to be successful, both the doctor and the patient must communicate effectively and work as a team. They need to be on the same page, so to speak, which happens less often than it should. A recent survey by TeleVox Software, which creates patient communication tools, found that 83 percent of patients don't follow the treatment plans their doctors recommend. Physicians put that number even higher—at 95 percent! In another study by *Consumer Reports,* nearly 700 doctors said their number-one complaint was failure by patients to follow medical advice and treatment recommendations. I have to admit, as much as I enjoy my profession, that is also my biggest frustration. Of course, I realize that patients have their fair share of complaints regarding doctors.

Why is there such a disconnect between doctors and patients? The reasons patients cited for their lack of follow-through included: not knowing enough about the condition or medication; frustration with side effects; feeling better and therefore believing the treatment is no longer needed; and not being able to afford it. These may be valid reasons for not following a doctor's orders, but instead of simply discontinuing treatment, they should be discussed with your physician in order to find solutions. In my opinion, developing a good rapport is a shared responsibility between both patients and physicians. So, perhaps, a better question might be: what can we do to improve the situation?

What to Expect from Your Doctor

The General Medical Council (GMC) states that doctors have a duty to create a partnership with their patients so that each party has an equal role in assessing the medical needs of the patient. That partnership must be based on openness, trust, and good communication. You also have a right to expect your physician to:

- Be polite, considerate, and honest.
- Treat you as an individual and with dignity.

- Respect your privacy and right to confidentiality.
- Provide support to care for yourself in order to improve and maintain your health.
- Encourage you to learn about your condition and use that information when you are making decisions about your care.
- Listen to you, ask for and respect your views, and respond to your concerns and preferences.
- Share information about your condition and treatment options in a way you can understand, including associated risks.
- Respond to your questions and keep you informed about the progress of your care.

When you are meeting with a physician for the first time, and as you continue to interact, you should ask yourself if he or she is adhering to this list. It's important to start the relationship off on the right foot.

Patient Responsibilities

Of course, communication is a two-way street. As the patient, you have some responsibilities, as well. You, too, must be open and honest. When I ask patients if they have been adhering to the migraine diet, for example, I would rather they confess to cheating than tell me what they think I want to hear. I can't make an accurate assessment without accurate data. You should also come prepared with as much information as possible about your condition. Keep an open mind and actively listen to the physician's advice. You might even want to take notes, if appropriate. Ask questions about any aspect of your condition or treatment you don't understand. Once you leave the office, keep your doctor informed of any problems, changes, side effects or progress that occurs. So, rather than simply discontinuing a medication because it causes unpleasant side effects, call the office and discuss the situation with your doctor. In other words, keep communications open and ongoing. And, by all means, follow your doctor's orders!

I would also add that, in order for any treatment to be effective, patients must be ready to understand and accept treatment. Sometimes when the diagnosis is difficult to hear, as in the case of life-changing or life-threatening illnesses, people need time to process the information and come to terms with it. The same thing can be said about treating headaches—you must be ready and willing to take the steps necessary to manage your condition. Since you are reading this book, I will assume you are tired of having headaches, looking for answers, and prepared to make a change. If headaches are interfering with your life; if you are missing work, school, or family functions; if you are afraid of making plans because you might get a headache; then it's time to develop a treatment plan. Let's start with your first doctor's appointment.

The Initial Visit

When you take your car in for repair, you want the vehicle to be making that mysterious clunking noise when you arrive so the mechanic can hear it firsthand. When it comes to headache disorders, the opposite is true. Most doctors would prefer you come to your first appointment when you are *not* having a headache, if possible. You'll be better able to provide accurate information and listen to your doctor when your head isn't throbbing with pain. Of course, the exception to this would be an injury or head trauma, or if you suddenly get a new, severe headache accompanied by fever or a stiff neck, in which case you should see a physician right away.

A headache consultation is typically a more lengthy appointment than normal, as it should delve into your medical history, your family's medical history, your headache history, all of your medications and treatments, your dietary and sleeping habits, and a review of your headache diary if you've been keeping one. You may also be asked to submit to certain lab tests.

It may seem like information overload, but gathering this data helps the doctor form a complete picture of you and your condition, as well as determining a baseline or level of "wellness." Remember, the goal is to treat not just your headaches, but you as an entire person. The more prepared you are, the more productive your visit will be. Before you go to this initial appointment, take some time to answer the following questions:

1. How many different types of headaches do you have, or is it just one type?

2. When did the headaches start—from childhood to present time?

3. Did the headaches begin after some accident or trauma to the head, or following a major life event, death in the family, etc.?

4. How often does the headache occur?

5. What does the pain feel like—throbbing, sharp, dull, squeezing, etc.?

6. Where is the pain located? Where does it start and/or travel to?

7. Are your present headaches becoming more severe?

8. Are they occurring more frequently?

9. Do your headaches wake you from sleep?

10. Is there anything you can identify that makes the headache worse, such as certain foods, drinks, activities, situations, etc.?

11. Can you tell when the headache is about to start? If so, what premonitory symptoms do you experience?

12. Do you feel depressed or anxious for several hours or a day before the headache begins?

13. Do you have any other symptoms along with your headache, such as nausea, vomiting, dizziness, sensitivity to light or sound, or tingling of the extremities?

14. When you get a headache, do you normally want to stop what you are doing and rest?

15. Does your headache become worse with activity?

16. How long do your headaches typically last?

17. What, if anything, makes your headaches better?

18. What makes them worse?

19. Do you have any other medical problems such as asthma, inhalant allergies, TMJ syndrome, IBS, irregular menstrual periods, palpitations of the heart or depression?

20. Are you taking any medications regularly, and if so, what are they? (Note: it's a good idea to make a list of all medications you are taking, including vitamins and OTC products. Be sure to write down the dosages and number of times a day or week you are taking the medications.)

21. What medications, if any, help the headaches, and what medications, if any, make them worse?

22. Does anyone else in your family have bad headaches?

23. Have you developed a new headache that is quite severe or one that is different than before?

24. Is it the worst headache you've had in your life?

25. Does your headache occur with fever?

26. Is your headache accompanied by a severely stiff, painful neck?

27. Do you have any neurological symptoms such as numbness on one side of your body, change in your reflexes, or loss or change of vision in one or both eyes?

28. Does your headache start when you awake in the morning and then get worse over a period of time?

29. Do your headaches coincide with your menstrual period?

30. What do you think is causing your headaches?

Again, this may seem like a lot of questions, but being prepared with as much information as possible prior to seeing your doctor will make the appointment go more smoothly and help him/her to make a more accurate diagnosis. Don't rely on your memory; write your answers down and bring them with you.

If you have been keeping a headache diary, bring that along.

Now that you've observed and described your headaches, think about how you feel in between attacks. Do you have problems sleeping? Do you feel anxious or depressed? Do you feel fatigued or foggy even when you are not having a headache?

The next step is to list any specific concerns or questions you may have. It's amazing how easily we forget what we wanted to ask the doctor as soon as he or she enters the examination room! If you come prepared with notes, you'll be sure to cover all the points you had in mind. Also, don't be afraid to voice your fears. If you are concerned that you have a brain tumor or aneurysm, for instance, let your doctor know. You should never be made to feel your concerns are irrational or unwarranted. Remember, honest communication is essential in this partnership.

Another tool that may be helpful for this initial visit is the Migraine Disability Assessment (MIDAS) questionnaire (see Appendix III). This measures the impact of your headaches, such as how much time you've lost due to headaches at work or school, as well as how your family, social, and leisure activities have been affected. The scores from this questionnaire can help your doctor determine which type of medications may be indicated.

Finally, I would recommend that you take a few moments to think about lifestyle issues. How much caffeine do you ingest each day? How many alcoholic beverages do you drink each week, particularly red wine and champagne? What other dietary triggers such as MSG, artificial sweeteners, and aged cheese, do you consume? Do you eat regular meals, including breakfast? How much exercise do you get each week? Do you go to bed

Let's Review:

- Open, honest communication is essential for an effective doctor-patient partnership.
- Making an accurate diagnosis is the first step in developing a treatment plan. To do that, you must participate in the process by taking the time to observe your headaches, and provide thorough and accurate information to your doctor.
- Use the resources in this book, such as the Headache Diary (Appendix I), the questions listed in this chapter, and the MIDAS questionnaire (Appendix III) to prepare for your appointment.
- Bring a list of questions to your initial visit, and be sure to communicate all concerns and fears with your doctor.

and wake up at approximately the same time each day? Are you a smoker? If so, are you willing to quit? Have an honest discussion with yourself regarding these issues and come prepared to discuss them with your doctor.

Follow-Up Appointments

Throughout this book, I have cautioned that treating headaches takes time and patience. Remember, migraines cannot be cured, but the condition can be managed. In fact, migraine is among the most successfully managed of all neurologic disorders. The key is knowledge. Over time, both you and your physician will gain knowledge about your particular condition, and using this information you will learn how to prevent headaches, as well as relieving them when they do occur. As you might expect, this will require more than one visit to your doctor.

Once a diagnosis is made, and a treatment plan is put in place, including lifestyle modifications and/or medications, it's very important to follow up with your physician on a regular basis. Often, these visits are brief and uninformative. To make them more productive, ask yourself the following questions, and be prepared to discuss the answers:

1. Has there been any change in my headaches (improvement or worsening), or in my general health since my last visit?

2. Have my headache patterns altered—become more or less frequent, more or less severe, longer or shorter in duration? (Bring your headache diary with you!)

3. Have I been following the migraine diet? Have I noticed any effect?

4. What other lifestyle changes have I made (exercise, stress reduction, etc.)? Have I noticed any effect?

5. Have I been taking my medication as directed? Is it working?

6. Have I experienced any side effects from the medication? If so, describe them.

7. Do I have trouble taking my medication or keeping it down due to nausea or stomach upset?

8. How quickly does the medication work to alleviate my headache once it begins?

9. How confident do I feel in my ability to manage my headaches now (in preventing them and treating them once a headache begins)?

This is also the time to ask any follow-up questions you may have regarding the treatment plan. Do you understand all aspects of the treatment? Do you know when and how to take your medications correctly? And, perhaps most importantly, what's next? If things are

> **Let's Review:**
> - Developing an effective treatment plan for migraine takes time and patience.
> - Follow-up visits with your physician are key to managing your headaches.
> - To make the most of these appointments, come prepared with information about changes in your headaches and your general health, as well as how lifestyle modifications and medications are working. A headache diary is very helpful.

improving, there may be no changes to the treatment plan, for the time being. Your doctor might not need to see you again for several months, unless there is a problem, to reassess your progress. However, if things have not improved, or become worse, it's time to discuss alternative strategies. Perhaps the dosage of your medication needs to be adjusted, or a new medication may be prescribed. Think of this process as a marathon, rather than a sprint. You may become tired or frustrated along the way, but the prize at the end is worth the effort.

When Treatment Fails

Over the years, there have been a small number of my headache patients that do not improve, even after exhausting all treatment options. Many of my fellow physicians agree that this is the most frustrating and disheartening situation we encounter. We begin to question ourselves: Do we fully understand and appreciate the magnitude or severity of these patients' headaches? Have we explored all possible treatment options? Are we missing some critical element? In some cases, we will never know the answers, but through experience we have identified a few possible explanations.

As mentioned earlier, when there is a lawsuit or disability claim involved, a patient may not get better because it's not in his or her best interest. Whether it's intentional or subconscious, the legalities interfere with the patient's motivation to respond to treatment. Even after the situation is resolved, some patients continue to have headaches because they have actually become dependent on them. For some, headaches elicit sympathy from family members, or provide an excuse for not working or participating in family responsibilities. Headaches become a type of crutch.

Another area of concern is when a patient is taking a narcotic on a regular basis for pain due to another condition, such as a back problem. The medication alleviates the back pain, but causes rebound headaches that are impossible to control. Abortive migraine medication does not seem to work well when a patient is already taking a narcotic or opioid. The vicious cycle of narcotics and rebound must be broken before the headaches can be relieved.

A more complex problem occurs when headaches are part of deeper emotional or psychological issues, such as post-traumatic stress disorder or chronic depression/anxiety. Ongoing depression can interfere with treatment, especially if it goes unrecognized and untreated. For some people, the feelings of stress, anxiety, depression or anger are so severe they actually resort to the headache to calm these intense emotions down or take the focus off the more debilitating condition. When the headache is relieved, the emotional issues resurface. In these cases, patients require psychiatric intervention.

You Can Win This Fight

Thankfully, most patients do not fall into any of these categories. Most of my patients are easy. They want reassurance that their disorder is benign, along with a treatment plan that relieves their headaches. The majority of them are also willing to make lifestyle changes and take their medication correctly. In fact, I am happy to say that most of my patients are success stories, which is very gratifying. Although I'd like to think I have some unique gift for curing headaches, I don't. The steps I've outlined in this book are really a common-sense approach to treating migraine based on years of experience. They have helped many people control their headaches and regain their lives—and they can help you, too. You've already taken the first step by reading this book. As you move forward, you can use the Treatment Plan Checklist (Appendix IV) to keep track of your progress.

In addition to the basics—stopping rebound, avoiding triggers, and preventing or derailing migraine with medication—I would like to add a few words of advice. Over the years, I have identified two attributes that make a person more likely to respond to treatment and achieve success: positive thinking and life balance. No matter how long it takes to find an effective treatment, maintaining a positive attitude can go a long way toward your progress. Tell yourself it can be done, and take a positive step forward each day. Finding a healthy balance in a busy life can be difficult, but it's not impossible. Patients who are able to balance work with play; exercise with relaxation; family time with time alone, and so on, are generally less anxious and better able to cope with life's demands. Achieving mental, physical, emotional, and spiritual balance can take a lifetime, but even the attempt can reduce stress and improve your well-being.

When all is said and done, *you* are the most important component in any treatment plan, including this one. Think of yourself as a boxer in training. Your opponent is migraine. I have equipped you with all the strategies and moves you need to win this fight. All you have to do is step into the ring and begin the first round. If you follow the steps I've outlined, I have every confidence that you can knock out headaches.

"Thank you for giving me my life back."

Let's end with a typical success story. Amy is a PhD psychologist with a ten-year history of severe incapacitating headaches. I have not seen Amy for quite a while, but I remember how much she was suffering when she first came to see me—and how skeptical she was regarding my advice. Following our first consultation, she went home and thought to herself, "This guy wants me to go to bed and get up at the same time every day, eat three meals day, and eliminate my Diet Cokes and coffee. Is he crazy? I have a husband who works seven days a week and five young children running around in all directions."

However, once Amy had some time to absorb this information, she thought it might have some merit. After all, she had been to six other physicians over the years and every treatment, thus far, had been unsuccessful. Her head continued to pound. And, if she was being honest with herself, she had to admit that she didn't sleep well, and was negligent regarding meals, often just grabbing a snack here or there. The caffeine was leaving her feeling wired, and she had no time for herself or anyone else. So, she said, "What the heck," and began taking the necessary steps to rid herself of headaches.

Amy stopped taking the OTC painkillers and made an effort to normalize her sleep patterns and eat regular meals. It took a great deal of willpower, but she managed to remove caffeine and artificial sweeteners from her diet, as well as foods that are known migraine triggers. She began taking a migraine medication as prescribed.

Slowly but surely, her debilitating headaches subsided. As the treatment began to work, she found that she actually slept better, had more energy during the day, and more time to do the things she used to enjoy.

Today, Amy is committed to the program and headache free. Sitting in my office for a follow-up visit, I notice how happy and bubbly she is as she talks about her family. On her way out, she stopped to say, "Thank you, Dr. Ruoff, for giving me my life back." I reminded her that, although I helped, it was really she who had knocked out the headaches. And you can, too.

Some Commonly Asked Questions and Answers

General

Are there any blood tests or other diagnostic tests to determine whether I have migraine headaches or not?

Unfortunately, no. Once a neurological exam is done to rule out any organic or secondary cause for your headaches, we rely on your medical history, a general physical exam, and information about your headache symptoms to make a diagnosis. That's why it's so important to provide as many facts as you can to your physician regarding the frequency and severity of your headaches, as well as the type of pain and possible triggers you've recognized. A headache diary can help you identify patterns, dietary issues, the effects of medication and other important clues.

Will I outgrow my migraines?

There is some evidence to suggest that as a person ages, both the frequency and severity of headaches decrease. Unfortunately, we can't tell you who will improve with age and who will continue to have headaches. Headaches associated with the menstrual cycle usually resolve after menopause.

Are my children destined to suffer from migraines?

Children of migraine sufferers have at least a 50% chance of developing the migraine syndrome themselves. Again, there is no way of knowing if your children will inherit migraines until they begin to exhibit symptoms. Keep in mind that migraines in children can differ greatly from those in adults (see chapter two). No one wants their children to suffer the pain of headaches, but they can be controlled using the program outlined in this book.

Can migraines be cured?

There is no cure for migraines, but they can be controlled. That's the whole idea behind this book—to help you take control of your migraine symptoms and maintain a good quality of life.

I don't get a premonitory aura or other pre-headache symptoms. Is it still a migraine if some of the headache phases are missing?

Yes. It's possible to have prodrome (the premonitory phase) with aura and have no headache, and then experience a postdrome or post-headache period. Every patient is different, and there are many possible combinations of symptoms that still classify the condition as migraine. You may have distinct premonitory symptoms that warn you of an impending headache, or none at all. You may have severe migraines without aura; or you could have no prodrome or aura, but have a headache that comes on in the postdrome phase. Remember, not all headaches are created equal.

I have had the same type of headache for many years, but now things are beginning to change. Should I be concerned?

Any change in your headaches, such as an increase in severity or location of pain, should be discussed with your physician. Though migraines can change over time, there is a possibility that you are developing another type of headache, which may be more serious and should be investigated thoroughly.

I have heard that migraine with aura can cause a stroke. Is this true?

It does happen, but it's extremely rare, and usually occurs in a person who has a predisposition towards stroke (a small portion of the population). For example, women, over 35 years of age, who take birth control pills and smoke tobacco, are at greater risk for stroke.

When I get my headaches, my hair and scalp are very sensitive—even my glasses hurt my nose and the sides of my head. Is this normal?

You are experiencing a condition called *cutaneous allodynia*, which is part of the migraine mechanism. The headache causes increased sensitivity in the nerve endings in certain areas of the face and head, which can be painful to the touch.

Diet/Lifestyle

After I saw the migraine prevention diet, I felt like there was nothing I could eat!

Take another look. There are actually many more foods and beverages *allowed* on the diet than restricted. The diet represents change, and change can be difficult. I understand that eliminating certain foods and beverages, particularly those you really enjoy, is not easy. However, it's the only way we can discover which dietary items aggravate your particular headaches. Not everyone reacts the same way to potential triggers. Keep in mind, the diet is much more restrictive in the beginning. After a few months, you can begin to add back items, *one at a time*, and see if they aggravate your headaches. Still, if you are prone to headaches, there are some things you may never be able to tolerate, such as caffeine.

My doctor said I shouldn't eat chocolate, but I can have a piece chocolate once in a while and it doesn't cause a headache. Is it really a trigger?

As we've discussed, triggers are cumulative. You may be able to have a piece of chocolate now and then without causing a headache. However, you don't want to have chocolate during your menstrual period, for example; or on a day when the barometer is rising or when you are under a lot of stress. And, washing that chocolate down with a glass of red wine is probably not be a good idea. It's only when the triggers exceed your migraine threshold that a headache is activated. Try not to overfill your glass!

Even though I can't have it, I crave chocolate. Why?

It's interesting to me that many patients will crave the particular food or beverage that is causing the most trouble with their headaches, whether it be caffeine, drinks with artificial sweeteners, or chocolate. Maybe it's just human nature to crave what we can't have. All I can say is it's probably not worth the pain. Try to find something else to satisfy the craving.

Ugh! Why do I always get a headache on the weekend when I'm ready to relax and have fun?

Like many people, you work hard all week and may have a stressful job, so it's natural to want to let off a little steam on the weekend. Sometimes, the release of tension or anxiety that you've been keeping bottled up all week is enough to trigger a headache. Often, though, it's the other weekend habits that lead to a headache: staying up later than usual and sleeping in (a disruption in sleep patterns); skipping meals; drinking too much red wine; fueling up with caffeine (which leads to withdrawal come Monday morning); or a combination of these common triggers.

Women's Issues

My headaches are associated with my menstrual cycle and are quite severe. Should I consider having a hysterectomy to solve my headache problem?

Absolutely not! It's a drastic treatment without a guarantee. While some patients may benefit from a hysterectomy, others will experience the same frequency and severity of headaches after the procedure. Still others end up with more pronounced headaches after surgery. There is no way to predict what the effect will be. In addition, a hysterectomy is a major surgery, which comes with its own risks and side effects, including the possible need for hormone replacement therapy, which can sometimes aggravate a headache problem.

The doctor put me on birth control pills and now my headaches are worse. Should I stop taking them?

Yes. Oral contraceptives are a fairly common migraine trigger. In fact, many women who suffer from migraines only during their menstrual period while taking birth control pills can put an end to their headaches simply by discontinuing the pills. If oral contraceptives are necessary, however, you may be able to switch to a different type. Birth control pills that have the same estrogen or progesterone content for the full 20-21 days, versus those that cause a gradual increase in the hormones, tend to be better tolerated. Also, formulas with smaller doses of estrogen may be less aggravating.

Why do my headaches go away when I'm pregnant?

Many women find that their migraines either improve or disappear completely during pregnancy due to the stabilization of hormones in the body (i.e., the lack of menstruation). Unfortunately, the headaches typically return to their usual pattern after pregnancy. A few unlucky women will experience worse headaches during pregnancy. It really depends on the individual and their particular migraine mechanism.

Treatment

What's the difference between abortive and preventive migraine medication?

Abortive medication is taken only when you have a migraine—ideally, at the first sign of a headache. It can either be a migraine-specific medication or an analgesic (painkiller) prescribed specifically to treat your headaches. Preventive medication is taken every day, whether you have a headache or not. It's designed to reduce the frequency and severity of your headaches on a long-term basis by raising the migraine threshold.

Do vitamins help prevent headaches?

Daily multi-vitamins and minerals are good for overall health, but have no proven effect on headaches. There are some studies that indicate that vitamins in very high potencies can actually aggravate headaches.

On the other hand, some vitamins and minerals might be helpful in reducing headaches. For instance, magnesium at dosages of 200–600 mg, riboflavin or vitamin B2 at dosages of 200–400 mg, and coenzyme Q10 at dosages of 100–200 mg, individually or in combination are beneficial to some patients.

Will a daily aspirin be helpful for headache control?

Several years ago, women's health studies demonstrated that a daily low-dose aspirin decreased headaches in patients by 15–20%. Taking a low-dose aspirin for cardiovascular reasons may also help decrease headaches in some patients.

I have tried several types of preventive medication for two or three weeks, and none of them worked. What can I do?

You need to give it a little more time. Depending on the type of medication, it can take up to three months for a preventive migraine drug to perform its function. It's important to gradually increase the dosage, starting low and working up to the level that is effective for your headache prevention. It takes time for the medication to get into your system and do its job.

If I developed rebound headaches from a certain medication, can I ever take it again?

Perhaps. If a general medication that is causing rebound headaches is discontinued, it may be reintroduced after several months, but only if it's taken infrequently (less than two times per week). Otherwise, you risk developing rebound again.

I have a friend who uses medicinal marijuana for chronic pain. Could it help my migraines?

To date, there are several studies that show marijuana is helpful for some migraine patients, though smoking seems to aggravate headaches. In some small antidotal studies, marijuana actually made the headaches worse, so it depends on the individual and their particular migraine mechanism.

I just want the pain to go away. Wouldn't it just be better if I took a strong narcotic to knock out my headaches?

Patients who rely on strong narcotics, especially on a daily basis, will develop rebound headaches, as well as a dependency on the drugs. Over time, they will need to increase the dosage and frequency of the medication to be effective. Many patients also develop "breakthrough headaches," even while on strong painkillers, therefore needing more and more medication. This creates a vicious cycle that is very difficult to break, and in many cases, the headaches become worse as time goes by. Patients who become addicted to narcotics may also require hospitalization to discontinue them.

Will wearing a copper bracelet or other type of "headache prevention" jewelry help?

There are no controlled studies that demonstrate the effectiveness of copper bracelets or other jewelry in treating headaches. There may be a placebo effect in some patients, however; if they believe the bracelet is working, they may actually experience fewer headaches. In general, I caution patients to be wary of any "miracle cures." If it sounds too good to be true, it usually is.

Appendix 1

Headache Diary

	Date	Headache		Severity (0-3 scale) 0=none; 1=mild; 2=moderate; 3=severe	Associated Migraine Symptoms 0=none; 1=nausea; 2=vomiting; 3=photophobia; 4=phonophobia	Disability (0-3 scale) 0=none; 1=mild; 2=moderate; 3=severe	Triggers	Miscellaneous
		Start Time	Stop Time					
Sunday								
Monday								
Tuesday								
Wednesday								
Thursday								
Friday								
Saturday								

Adapted from Abbott Laboratories, August 1996

Appendix II

Complete and review with your doctor on your next visit.

Hamilton Anxiety Rating Scale

Item	Rating	Item	Rating
Anxious Mood		**Somatic (Sensory)**	
Worries, anticipation of the worst, fearful anticipation, irritability		Tinnitus, blurring of vision, hot and cold flushes, feelings of weakness, picking sensation	
Tension		**Cardiovascular Symptoms**	
Feelings of tension, fatigability, startle response, moved to tears easily, trembling, feelings of restlessness, inability to relax		Tachycardia, palpitations, pain in chest, throbbing of vessels, fainting feelings, missing beat	

0=None
1=Mild
2=Moderate
3=Severe
4=Very Severe

Fear			Respiratory Symptoms		
Of dark, of strangers, of being left alone, of animals, of traffic, of crowds			Pressure or constriction in chest, choking feelings, sighing, dyspnea		
Insomnia			**Gastrointestinal Symptoms**		
Difficulty falling asleep, broken sleep, unsatisfying sleep and fatigue upon waking, dreams, nightmares, night terrors			Difficulty in swallowing, wind, abdominal pain, burning sensations, abdominal fullness, nausea, vomiting, borborygmi, looseness of bowels, loss of weight, constipation		
Intellectual (Cognitive)			**Genitourinary Symptoms**		
Difficulty concentrating, poor memory			Frequency of micturition, urgency of micturition, amenorrhea, menorrhagia, development of frigidity, premature ejaculation, loss of libido, impotence		

Depressed Mood			Autonomic Symptoms		
Loss of interest, lack of pleasure in hobbies, depression, early waking, diurnal swing			Dry mouth, flushing, pallor, tendency to sweat, giddiness, tension headache, raising of hair		
Behavior at Interview			**Somatic (Muscular)**		
Fidgeting, restlessness or pacing, tremor of hands, furrowed brow, strained face, sighing or rapid respiration, facial pallor, swallowing, belching, brisk tendon jerks, dilated pupils, exophthalmos			Pains and aches, twitchings, stiffness, myoclonic jerks, grinding of teeth, unsteady voice, increased muscular tone		

1989, MeadJohnson Pharmaceuticals, Bristol-Meyers Company, Evansville, IN USA

Appendix III

Migraine Disability Assessment

This questionnaire is used to determine the level of pain and disability caused by your headaches and helps your doctor find the best treatment for you.

Please answer the following questions about all your headaches over the last **3 months**. Write your answer in the box next to each question. Write zero if you did not do the activity in the last **3 months**.

1) On how many days in the last 3 months did you miss work or school because of your headaches? *(If you do not attend work or school enter zero in the box).*

   □□ Days

2) How many days in the last 3 months was your productivity at work or school reduced by half or more because of your headaches? *(Do not include days you counted in question 1 where you missed work or school. If you do not attend work or school enter zero in the box).*

   □□ Days

3) On how many days in the last 3 months did you not do household work because of your headaches?

   □□ Days

4) How many days in the last 3 months was your productivity in household work reduced by half or more because

of your headaches? (Do not include days you counted in question 3 where you did not do household work).

☐☐ Days

5) On how many days in the last 3 months did you miss family, social, or leisure activities because of your headaches?

☐☐ Days

Questions 1-5 total: _____

Midas Grade	Definition	Midas Score
I	Little or no disability	0-5
II	Mild disability	6-10
III	Moderate disability	11-20
IV	Severe disability	21+

A) On how many days in the last 3 months did you have a headache? (If headache lasted more than 1 day, count each day).

☐☐ Days

B) On a scale of 0-10, on average how painful were these headaches? (Where 0=no pain at all, and 10=pain that is as bad as it can be).

☐☐ Days

Appendix IV

Developing Your Personal Headache Treatment Plan

As you read through this book, use this checklist to start developing your own headache treatment plan. Each step you complete in the process is one step closer to ridding yourself of headache pain and regaining your life!

I. Understanding My Headaches

_____ I have kept a headache diary for at least one month.

Have any patterns emerged? _____

I have identified the following potential triggers:

_____

_____

II. Medications

If you were taking pain medications, either OTC or prescription, for your headaches without relief:

_____ With the guidance of a physician, I have discontinued using painkillers in order to prevent rebound headaches.

_____ I have talked with my physician about alternative migraine medications.

If you have tried lifestyle modifications for several months without relief:

_____ I have talked with my physician about acute migraine medications to be used in conjunction with lifestyle modifications.

If you have been using acute migraine medications without relief:

____ I have talked with my physician about preventive migraine medications to be used in conjunction with lifestyle modifications.

III. Lifestyle Modifications

____ I have eliminated known migraine triggers from my diet, including caffeine, MSG, alcohol (particularly red wine and champagne), chocolate, and artificial sweeteners.

____ I have followed the migraine prevention diet for at least 2 months.

Have you noticed any changes? _____

____ I have regulated my sleep patterns by going to bed and waking up at the same time every day, and making my bedroom more restful.

____ I have begun (with the advice of a physician) an exercise routine, and have exercised regularly for at least six weeks.

____ I have practiced the neck exercises on pages 97–98 daily to reduce muscle tension in my neck and shoulders, and improve flexibility.

____ I have incorporated a stretching-type exercise into my routine, such as yoga, Pilates or Tai Chi.

____ I have adopted some stress-reduction techniques, such as meditation, massage, relaxing in a quiet room for 15–20 minutes, keeping a journal, delegating chores, etc.

____ I have "headache proofed" my house, including reducing glare and fluorescent lights, using dimmers, eliminating overpowering scents, claiming a quiet space for myself, etc.

_____ If you have abnormal muscle tightness or spasms: I have consulted with a physical therapist.

_____ I have adjusted my work space to be ergonomically correct.

Resources

National Headache Foundation: www.headaches.org/

American Headache Society (for patients or physicians): www.americanheadachesociety.org/

Committee for Headache Education (ACHE-for patients): www.achenet.org/

To order vitamins: www.preventyourheadache.com/, 269-375-1700

Index

Genetic influence in bipolar
 depression 157
Giant cell temporal arteritis
 in seniors 86–87
 symptoms of 80

Hamilton Anxiety Rating
 Scale 160, **206–208**
Happiness, methods for pro-
 moting 112–113
Headache consultation 181
 follow-up appointments. *See*
  Follow-up appointments
 initial visit to doctor. *See* Initial visit to doctor
 treatment failure 189
  abortive migraine medication 190
  identifying causes of 190
  lawsuit/disability claim
   190
  patient's motivation 190
  psychological issues 191
Headache diary, keeping 185,
 195
 advantages of 92
 associated symptoms 91
 date and time of headache
  91
 dietary triggers 91, 102
 feelings 91
 format for **205**
 improving condition 92
 pain intensity 91
 timing, duration, and severity of headaches 91
 triggers and patterns 90
 women sufferers 92
Headache disorder 15

Headache management 11,
 55. *See also* Headache
 consultation
 alternative treatment. *See*
  Alternative medicine
 basic steps of 19, 20
 cautionary sign in 41
 changes in home for
  110–111
 copper bracelets effectiveness in 204
 by dietary changes 46
 by lifestyle modifica-
  tions. *See* Lifestyle
  modifications
 migraine triggers. *See*
  Migraine triggers
 30 minutes of rest and quiet
  111, 113
 success stories of 193–194
 systematic approach to
  148–149
Headache patients
 frustration among 17, 18
 multiple diagnoses of 62
Headaches 9
 causes of 15
  questions about 19
 changeable nature of 62
 changes in patterns if 197
 control by lifestyle changes
  32–33
 control of 131–133
 development phases
  localized pain 51
  migraine diary 53
  mild phase 50–51
  moderate-to-severe phase
   51–52

Vasodilators as migraine triggers 45
Vitamins, managing headaches with
  riboflavin 117, 202
  side effects of 201
  vitamin B2 202
  vitamin B12 118
Vomiting, severe/recurrent
  associated with migraine 57–58
  treatment of 140–141, **141**

Wafers. *See* Oral disintegrating tablets

Weather changes, headache caused by 74
  case study of 76–77
Weight loss and migraine prevention diet 110
Women, headaches in. *See* Headaches in women
Work balance 192

Yeast-risen baked goods 40
Yoga 114–115

Gary E. Ruoff, MD

Dr. Ruoff is one of the founders of the Westside Family Medical Center in Kalamazoo, Michigan, and presently serves as Director of Clinical Research at that facility. Dr. Ruoff is also Clinical Professor of Family Practice at Michigan State University College of Medicine in East Lansing. He completed his undergraduate work at St. Peters College in Jersey City, New Jersey, and earned his medical degree from Loyola University in Chicago, Illinois. Dr. Ruoff is certified by the American Board of Family Practice and the Board of Headache Management. He has authored over 90 articles, abstracts, and monographs in various specialties of medicine. Dr. Ruoff is very active in presenting research papers as well as lectures on both the national and international levels and has received numerous awards for his work. He is past President of the Michigan Academy of Family Physicians and served as a member of the Education Commission Research Committee and aspects of the Scientific Assembly Committee of the American Academy of Family Physicians. He also served as the Michigan delegate to the American Academy of Family Physicians. In addition, Dr. Ruoff is very involved in the teaching of students, residents, and physicians.